DOSAGE CALCULATIONS
IN SI UNITS

FOURTH EDITION

DOSAGE CALCULATIONS IN SI UNITS

FOURTH EDITION

MAUREEN OSIS RN, MN

Nurse Consultant
Osis Consulting Services Ltd.

Adjunct Assistant Professor, Faculty of Nursing
University of Calgary

Information Division
United States Pharmacopeia (USP)

Committee of Revision: Gerontology
Expert Committee Member

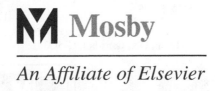 Mosby

An Affiliate of Elsevier

ELSEVIER
MOSBY

FOURTH EDITION
Copyright © 2003 Elsevier Canada, a division of Reed Elsevier Canada Ltd.

A Note to the Reader

The author and publisher have made every attempt to check dosages for accuracy. Because the science of pharmacology is continually advancing, the knowledge base continues to expand. Therefore, we recommend that the reader always check product information for changes in dosage or administration before administering any medication.

National Library of Canada Cataloguing in Publication Data

Osis, M. (Maureen)
    Dosage calculation in SI units

4th ed.
Accompanied by a CD-ROM containing 650 interactive questions that are self-scoring.
Includes index.
ISBN 0-920513-37-9

    1. Drugs—Dosage. 2. Pharmaceutical arithmetic. I. Title.

RS578.0754 2002   615'.14'01513   C2002-901045-4

Acquisitions Editor: Ann Millar
Developmental Editor: Liz Radojkovic
Production Editors: Gil Adamson/Shefali Mehta
Permissions Editor: Terri Rothman
Production Coordinator: Kimberly Sullivan
Copyeditor: Susan Harrison
Cover Design: Rivet Art + Design
Interior Design: Liz Harasymczuk
Page Composition: Carolyn Sebestyen
Typesetting: Heidy Lawrance Associates
Printing and Binding: King Printing Co., Inc.

Elsevier Canada
420 Main Street East, Suite 636, Milton, ON, Canada L9T 5G3
Phone: 416-644-7053

14 15 16 17   21 20 19 18 17

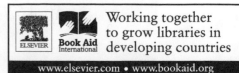

To all my past, present, and future nursing colleagues
who strive for safe and competent care.

Preface

Dosage Calculations in SI Units, Fourth Edition, offers you the opportunity to learn the skills required to calculate medication dosages, both simple and complex, in a variety of settings.

By learning how to calculate and to administer medications safely, you are investing in yourself and your ability to understand and accurately deliver medications. *Dosage Calculations in SI Units* helps you to achieve both accuracy and confidence.

▶ FEATURES OF THE FOURTH EDITION

This completely revised edition of *Dosage Calculations* provides the following features:

- The content is presented in an engaging writing style and an appealing format.
- A self-assessment test determines your comprehension of basic arithmetic skills.
- The book progresses from simple to more complex concepts.
- Each module presents the concepts in a clear, concise, easy-to-understand manner.
- Examples illustrate the concepts, followed by exercises containing many questions taken directly from clinical areas in both a rural and a large urban setting. The exercises are designed to test your comprehension and competency in the skill.
- Exercises present problems from a variety of perspectives and include novelty to encourage the practitioner to read carefully and approach all problems with attention.
- You can practise the concept you have just learned and then check your answers against the answer guide at the back of the book. Mastery of each concept is ensured by requiring a score of 100% on the post-test for each module.
- Post-tests at the end of each module evaluate progress and learning comprehension.
- Each module provides a variety of examples and exercises to simulate the clinical field as practitioners do dosage calculations in numerous settings.
- The content is focused on realistic, clinically relevant information.
- You are frequently encouraged to develop good habits for safe practice.
- Critical Point boxes highlight procedural concerns that you may encounter in practice.
- Case Studies are presented to illustrate realistic clinical situations.
- Drug labels from Canadian pharmaceutical companies acquaint you with the types of labels you will encounter in clinical practice.

Many of the changes to the fourth edition of *Dosage Calculations* were based on feedback from readers and reviewers. Some modules have been reorganized to include coverage of calculations for both pediatric and geriatric medications, and the critical care information is enhanced and located in a separate module for easy reference.

Tables summarizing the "Conversion of SI Units and Subunits" for "Units and Subunits" and a list of commonly used medication abbreviations are printed on the inside front cover of the book for quick reference. Four appendices appear at the end of the book: (1) Approximate Equivalents among Systems of Measurement; (2) Temperature Conversions; (3) Brand Names in Canada, Australia, and the United States; and (4) Problem-Solving Approach.

This fourth edition includes an interactive CD-ROM that contains a set of 50 questions for each of the 10 modules in the book. Each question provides a rationale for the correct answer. The 500 new questions are designed to help you learn the essential skills of dosage calculations. In addition to the 500 supplementary questions, the CD-ROM contains four comprehensive post-tests that cover material from each module. The post-tests are designed to evaluate your mastery of the concepts presented in the book. You will be challenged to use basic mathematical skills, abbreviations, various units of drug measurements, drug labels and tables, clinical scenarios, and common sense. Instructions on how to install the CD-ROM can be found on the face of the CD.

▶ HOW TO USE THIS BOOK

To the Student

It is best to proceed through the modules in sequence and be certain you are competent using ratio and proportion before attempting calculations. Develop a habit of safe practice — always check your answers intuitively (does it make sense?) and then be sure to validate your answers.

To International Students

This book was written by a Canadian, but SI units are a truly international system.

To the Nursing Instructor

I have designed this book to be used by the student in the classroom, in the laboratory, for clinical learning, or as an independent learning guide. Modules 1 to 6 are ideal for helping to reinforce information and to prepare students for lectures and laboratory demonstrations that introduce medication administration. Modules 7 to 10 provide more complex and specialized information that will be relevant to the more advanced nursing student.

To Other Instructors

In this age of change in health care, there is greater demand for more diverse health care professionals to be able to administer medication. This book is appropriate for many diverse groups. For example, licensed practical nurses will find Modules 1 to 5 useful as a foundation for oral administration. Furthermore, this book has been reviewed by a pharmacist to ensure that it is appropriate for pharmacy technicians.

▶ ACKNOWLEDGEMENTS

Many individuals reviewed the third edition and provided valuable suggestions for this new edition of *Dosage Calculations*. In particular I would like to thank the following:

Sally Corby, BN, Instructor, Red River College and the University of Manitoba
Marilynn Gillies, RN, BN, MA, Instructor, Dawson College
Barbara Jungmann, RN, for her contribution of common calculations in a rural setting
Lori Labatte, RN, BSc, BEd, Instructor, SIAST
Elizabeth Richard, RN, MN, Instructor, Grande Prairie Regional College

Margaret D. Seymour, RN, BN, Community Nursing Instructor, Medicine Hat College
Lee Wallace, RN, for her contribution of common calculations in an urban setting
Anna Wilson, RN, BScN, Professor, Fanshawe College
Joanne Wladyka, MScN, Professor, Seneca College
Leanne Wyrostok, RN, MN, Nursing Skills Clinician, University of Calgary

I would also like to thank the following companies for allowing the reproduction of
medication labels and various types of medication packaging systems:

Abbott Laboratories Limited, Montreal, Quebec
Baxter Corporation, Toronto, Ontario
Bioniche Pharma Group, London, Ontario
Eli Lilly Canada, Inc., Scarborough, Ontario
GlaxoSmithKline Inc., Mississauga, Ontario
Leo Pharma Inc., Thornhill, Ontario
Manrex Limited, Winnipeg, Manitoba
Novartis Pharmaceuticals Canada Inc., Dorval, Quebec
Novopharm Limited, Toronto, Ontario
Pharmacia Canada Inc., Mississauga, Ontario
Schering Canada Inc., Pointe-Claire, Quebec
Trianon Laboratories Inc., Blainville, Quebec
WellSpring Pharmaceutical Canada Corp., Oakville, Ontario

And I would especially like to thank my family, Imants, Andrew, Jody, Makenna, Lara,
and Sean for support and laughter throughout the process.

—Maureen Osis

Contents

Module 1 provides the opportunity for you to assess your skills in basic arithmetic, to analyze any areas of weakness you may have because you have not used arithmetic lately, and to review the concepts, if necessary. Basic arithmetic skills include addition, subtraction, multiplication, and division of whole numbers, decimal numbers, and fractions. These are the skills needed for dosage calculations — even complex calculations. Many students and novice health care professionals are anxious about calculating dosages, and it is reasonable to have a certain degree of caution and concern. You should want to "get it right." This book emphasizes that you can get it right, with practice and persistence, by using a step-by-step approach. For some individuals, this responsibility will be seen as an easy one because they like math and enjoy balancing their chequebooks each month. For others, who describe themselves as "math challenged," the task may appear daunting. You do not want to hear that it is easy, but you do need to hear that it is certainly possible for you to become self-confident and competent.

Here are some hints that you may find helpful:

- Use this book and other opportunities such as labs, practice exams, and classes to master the basic skills. Be sure that you understand the concept; don't just memorize the solution. Think of the joke "How do you get to Carnegie Hall? Practise, practise, practise." This book will give you lots of opportunity to practise until you understand each concept.

- Be aware of your attitude toward problem solving and applying arithmetic skills; being anxious can contribute to insecurity and mistakes, which, in turn, can make you feel more anxious. Change the negative self-talk from a self defeating message, for example, "I can't do math," to a more positive approach, such as "I can learn to use my intuition and my reasoning to solve the problem."

- Look for and accept additional help if you need it. There are different ways to solve problems, and someone else may have an approach that works for you. For example, you may meet instructors or preceptors who prefer to use a formula for dosage calculations because they learned this approach and have developed confidence in using it. Other instructors or preceptors may be more comfortable using ratio and proportion to do the calculation. Find the approach that works best for you.

- Don't let others rush you; it is accuracy, not speed, that is important.

- Don't think that you have to master everything at once. As you proceed through the book you will learn to do the following:
  - Set up proportion statements.
  - Use proportion for dosage calculations.
  - Use formulas for dosage calculations.
  - Use problem solving for dosage calculations.
  - Understand systems of measurement and convert among them.
  - Interpret medication labels and understand dosage forms.
  - Calculate medications in solid forms, such as tablets and capsules, and in liquid forms.

- When you have mastered the basics, you will move on to more challenging situations, such as the following:
  - Preparation and calculation of intravenous infusions
  - Mixing medications in one syringe
  - Following dosage protocols
  - Performing calculations unique to pediatric and geriatric patients
- Finally, you will have the opportunity to do the more complex calculations that occur in critical care settings, such as titrating intravenous medication flow rates.

Now it's time to check your current skills; complete the self-assessment test on page 3.

▶ WHOLE NUMBERS, FRACTIONS, DECIMAL NUMBERS, AND PERCENTS

Complete the following test to assess your skills in basic arithmetic. Correct your answers by using the answer guide starting on page 192. Each correct answer has a value of 1 mark. A score of 100% means you are ready to proceed to Module 2. If you do not achieve 100%, review the relevant sections of Module 1 and write the post-test. If your score is less than 100% on the post-test, you should obtain remedial assistance, which is beyond the scope of this book.

PART I

Whole Numbers

Perform the operation shown.

1. $842 + 679$
2. $1793 + 456$
3. $547 + 79$
4. $182 + 453$

5. $677 - 546$
6. $1799 - 610$
7. $942 - 864$
8. 328×42

9. 762×51
10. 4422×11
11. 876×13
12. $48 \div 12 =$

13. $78 \div 13 =$
14. $125 \div 25 =$
15. $1246 \div 14 =$

Your Score: /15 = %

PART II

Fractions

Perform the operation shown. Simplify where necessary.

1. $\frac{4}{12} + \frac{3}{9} =$
2. $\frac{1}{7} + \frac{5}{14} =$
3. $\frac{2}{4} + \frac{6}{9} =$
4. $\frac{2}{3} + 1 =$

5. $\frac{14}{22} - \frac{6}{10} =$
6. $\frac{3}{4} - \frac{16}{30} =$
7. $\frac{1}{2} - \frac{1}{8} =$
8. $9\frac{1}{3} - \frac{7}{12} =$

9. $1\frac{1}{9} - \frac{6}{10} =$
10. $\frac{1}{3} \times \frac{5}{8} =$
11. $\frac{3}{4} \times \frac{1}{16} =$
12. $3\frac{1}{5} \times \frac{2}{3} =$

13. $\frac{5}{8} \times \frac{1}{2} =$
14. $12 \times \frac{3}{5} =$
15. $\frac{7}{10} \times \frac{1}{3} =$
16. $\frac{9}{12} \div \frac{3}{4} =$

3

17. $\dfrac{4}{10} \div \dfrac{3}{5} =$ 18. $1\dfrac{1}{16} \div \dfrac{2}{8} =$ 19. $\dfrac{3}{8} \div \dfrac{1}{2} =$ 20. $\dfrac{2}{3} \div \dfrac{4}{9} =$

Change these improper fractions to mixed or whole numbers.

21. $\dfrac{52}{4}$ 22. $\dfrac{27}{5}$ 23. $\dfrac{47}{7}$

24. $\dfrac{86}{6}$ 25. $\dfrac{134}{11}$

Find the lowest common denominator.

26. $\dfrac{1}{2}$ and $\dfrac{2}{3}$ 27. $\dfrac{5}{8}$ and $\dfrac{3}{5}$ 28. $\dfrac{1}{6}$ and $\dfrac{1}{9}$

29. $\dfrac{1}{3}$ and $\dfrac{4}{7}$ 30. $\dfrac{1}{4}$ and $\dfrac{3}{16}$

Simplify these fractions to their lowest terms.

31. $\dfrac{12}{32}$ 32. $\dfrac{18}{42}$ 33. $\dfrac{25}{140}$

34. $\dfrac{16}{48}$ 35. $\dfrac{15}{32}$

State whether the following expressions are proper fractions, improper fractions, or mixed numbers.

36. $1\dfrac{1}{18}$ 37. $\dfrac{23}{14}$ 38. $\dfrac{6}{7}$

39. $\dfrac{1}{4}$ 40. $\dfrac{33}{10}$

Equivalent Fractions

Express each fraction as an equivalent fraction.

41. $\dfrac{1}{3} = \dfrac{?}{9}$ 42. $\dfrac{6}{2} = \dfrac{48}{?}$ 43. $\dfrac{1}{5} = \dfrac{5}{?}$

State whether the following expressions are equivalent fractions. (State *yes* or *no*.)

44. $\dfrac{3}{16} = \dfrac{9}{64}$ 45. $\dfrac{4}{26} = \dfrac{16}{104}$

Your Score: /45   =   %

PART III

Decimal Numbers

1. Write *one-quarter* in correct decimal format.

2. Write *one-half* in correct decimal format.

Rounding Decimal Numbers

Round the following decimal numbers to the nearest tenth.

3. 1.246   4. 1.09   5. 7.14

Round the following decimal numbers to the nearest hundredth.

6. 9.743   7. 15.547   8. 2.008

For each of the following pairs, choose the correct way of writing the decimal numbers.

9. 0.25   or   0.250   10. 0.2   or   .2   11. 1.0   or   1

Arithmetic of Decimal Numbers

Perform the operation shown.

12. $2.73 + 5.28 =$ 13. $0.71 + 0.24 + 5.6 =$ 14. $2.6 + 1.09 + 4.33 =$

15. $0.9 + 1.1 + 2.6 =$ 16. $9 - 2.4 =$ 17. $7.4 - 4.6 =$

18. $9.2 - 7.8 =$ 19. $5.1 - 0.9 =$ 20. $0.125 - 0.055 =$

21. $0.7 \times 10 =$ 22. $0.5 \times 1000 =$ 23. $0.1 \times 1 =$

24. $0.5 \times 100 =$ 25. $0.1 \times 0.1 =$

Complete the operation. Round each answer to the nearest tenth.

26. $3.6 \div 0.12 =$ 27. $44.02 \div 6.2 =$ 28. $2.5 \div 1.25 =$

29. $6.448 \div 1.24 =$ 30. $2.86 \div 1.3 =$

Converting Fractions, Decimal Numbers, and Percents

Convert these fractions into decimal numbers. Round each answer to the nearest hundredth.

31. $\dfrac{1}{6}$ 32. $1\dfrac{3}{5}$ 33. $\dfrac{3}{8}$

34. $\dfrac{18}{24}$ 35. $\dfrac{2}{16}$

Convert the following expressions into fractions. Simplify each answer to its lowest terms.

36. 0.7   37. 0.32   38. 1.25

39. 0.02   40. 1.01

41. Which of the following expressions is the smallest?

1.01   or   0.01   or   0.001

42. Which of the following expressions is the largest?

2.4   or   2.7   or   2.95   or   2.9

Convert fractions, decimal numbers, and percents in the following table using the given information. Follow the example given in the first line of the table. Express fractions in their lowest terms.

Fraction	Decimal Number	Percent
$\frac{1}{4}$	0.25	25%
(43)	0.9	(44)
$1\frac{3}{4}$	(45)	(46)
(47)	(48)	64%
(49)	0.004	(50)

Your Score:	/50 =	%

Total Score

Part I: Whole Numbers: /15 = _____%
Part II: Fractions: /45 = _____%
Part III: Decimal Numbers: /50 = _____%

Did you achieve 100% on each part?

YES — Proceed to Module 2.

NO — Analyze your areas of weakness and review the relevant sections of Module 1; then write the post-test.

Whole Numbers, Fractions, Decimal Numbers, and Percents

▶ MODULE TOPICS

- Fractions
  - Definitions
  - Types of fractions
  - Changing improper fractions and mixed numbers
  - Arithmetic of fractions
- Decimal numbers
  - Definitions
  - Rules for writing decimal numbers
  - Rounding decimal numbers
  - Arithmetic of decimal numbers
  - Converting fractions and decimal numbers
- Percents
  - Converting fractions, decimal numbers, and percents

▶ INTRODUCTION

This module provides a brief review of basic arithmetic skills of whole numbers, fractions, decimal numbers, and percents. This allows you the opportunity to assess your skills and to then decide whether you want to complete the entire module or do those sections that address your areas of weakness. Because these arithmetic skills are used time and again in the calculation of drug doses, you should master these skills before proceeding to other modules. If you do not have accuracy and confidence in this area, you are encouraged to obtain remedial assistance, which is beyond the scope of this book.

▶ FRACTIONS

Definitions

The word *fraction* is from the Latin *fractus*, meaning *broken*. A fraction is a number that represents a part of a whole unit.

Example: $\dfrac{3}{4}$

The *numerator* is the top value. The *denominator* is the bottom value.

Example: $\dfrac{3}{4} \begin{array}{l} \rightarrow \text{numerator} \\ \rightarrow \text{denominator} \end{array}$

Types of Fractions

Proper fraction: a fraction in which the numerator is smaller in value than the denominator.

Example: $\dfrac{1}{3}$

Improper fraction: a fraction in which the numerator is greater in value than the denominator.

Example: $\dfrac{4}{3}$

Mixed number: a unit that contains a whole number and a fraction.

Example: $1\dfrac{1}{3}$

Equivalent fractions: two or more fractions that have the same value but are expressed in different numbers. When the numerator and denominator are multiplied by the same number, the value of the fraction does not change. Likewise, both terms of a fraction can be divided by the same number without changing the value of the fraction. This is an important principle in the arithmetic of fractions. Many mathematical operations with fractions require expanding and reducing.

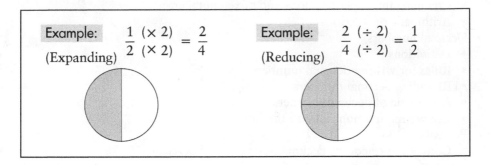

Example: $\dfrac{1\ (\times 2)}{2\ (\times 2)} = \dfrac{2}{4}$ (Expanding)

Example: $\dfrac{2\ (\div 2)}{4\ (\div 2)} = \dfrac{1}{2}$ (Reducing)

Lowest term: a fraction in which the numerator and the denominator are reduced to the lowest possible value by dividing the denominator and the numerator by the same number.

NOTE: Fractions must be simplified or expressed in lowest terms. See the example on page 9.

Example: $\dfrac{1}{2}$ is expressed in its lowest terms.

$\dfrac{2}{4}$ is not expressed in its lowest terms.

To simplify a fraction: 1. Divide both the numerator and the denominator by the same number.

2. Place the new value of the numerator over the new value of the denominator.

$$\dfrac{2}{4} = \dfrac{?}{?}$$

$$\dfrac{2 \ (\div 2)}{4 \ (\div 2)} = \dfrac{1}{2}$$

Changing Improper Fractions and Mixed Numbers

To change an improper fraction to a mixed number, divide the numerator by the denominator.

Example: $\dfrac{4}{3} = ?$

$$4 \div 3 = 1\dfrac{1}{3}$$

To change a mixed number to an improper fraction:

1. Multiply the whole number by the denominator.
2. Add the numerator to the product.
3. Place the sum over the denominator.

Example: $5\dfrac{1}{3} = ?$

$$5 \times 3 = 15$$

$$15 + 1 = 16$$

$$\dfrac{16}{3}$$

Arithmetic of Fractions

Adding fractions

To add fractions with the same denominator:

1. Add the numerators.
2. Place the sum over the denominator.
3. Simplify if necessary.

Example: $\dfrac{1}{5} + \dfrac{2}{5} = ?$

$$1 + 2 = 3$$

$$\dfrac{3}{5}$$

To add fractions with unlike denominators:

1. Find the common denominator. This is the smallest whole number that the denominators of the two or more fractions will divide into evenly. You can find the lowest common denominator by trial and error.

2. Convert each fraction to an equivalent fraction using the common denominator.

3. Add the numerators, and place the sum over the common denominator.

4. Simplify the answer.

Example: $\dfrac{1}{2} + \dfrac{2}{3} = ?$

Find the common denominator; both 2 and 3 divide evenly into 6.

Convert: $\dfrac{1\,(\times 3)}{2\,(\times 3)} = \dfrac{3}{6}$

$\dfrac{2\,(\times 2)}{3\,(\times 2)} = \dfrac{4}{6}$

Add: $\dfrac{3}{6} + \dfrac{4}{6} = \dfrac{3+4}{6} = \dfrac{7}{6}$

Simplify: $\dfrac{7}{6} = 1\dfrac{1}{6}$

Subtracting fractions

To subtract fractions that have the same denominator:

1. Subtract the numerators.

2. Place the answer over the denominator.

3. Simplify if necessary.

Example: $\dfrac{3}{4} - \dfrac{1}{4} = ?$

$3 - 1 = 2$

$\dfrac{2}{4} = \dfrac{1}{2}$

To subtract fractions with unlike denominators:

1. Find the common denominator. This is the smallest whole number that the denominators of the two (or more) fractions will divide into evenly.

2. Convert each fraction to an equivalent fraction using the common denominator.

3. Subtract the numerators and place the difference over the common denominator.

4. Simplify if necessary.

Example: $\dfrac{5}{6} - \dfrac{3}{8} = ?$

Find the common denominator; both 6 and 8 divide evenly into 24.

Convert: $\dfrac{5}{6} = \dfrac{?}{24} \quad \dfrac{5\,(\times 4)}{6\,(\times 4)} = \dfrac{20}{24}$

Convert: $\dfrac{3}{8} = \dfrac{?}{24} \quad \dfrac{3\,(\times 3)}{8\,(\times 3)} = \dfrac{9}{24}$

Subtract: $\dfrac{20-9}{24} = \dfrac{11}{24}$

Simplify: $\dfrac{11}{24}$ is expressed in its lowest terms.

Adding and subtracting mixed numbers

To add or subtract mixed numbers:

1. Convert the mixed number to an improper fraction.

2. Follow the steps outlined for addition and subtraction of fractions.

Example: $1\dfrac{1}{3} + \dfrac{3}{4} = ?$

Convert the mixed number:

$$1\dfrac{1}{3} \text{ is } \dfrac{4}{3}$$

Find the common denominator; 12 is evenly divided by both 3 and 4.

Convert: $\dfrac{4\,(\times 4)}{3\,(\times 4)} = \dfrac{16}{12}$

Convert: $\dfrac{3\,(\times 3)}{4\,(\times 3)} = \dfrac{9}{12}$

$$\dfrac{16+9}{12} = \dfrac{25}{12}$$

Convert to a mixed number:

$$\dfrac{25}{12} = 2\dfrac{1}{12}$$

Example: $2 - \dfrac{1}{2} = ?$

Convert the whole number to a fraction:

$$2 = \dfrac{2}{1}$$

Find the common denominator: 2

Convert: $\dfrac{2\,(\times 2)}{1\,(\times 2)} = \dfrac{4}{2}$

Subtract: $\dfrac{4-1}{2} = \dfrac{3}{2}$

Convert to a mixed number:

$$\dfrac{3}{2} = 1\dfrac{1}{2}$$

To add or subtract mixed numbers, you may also follow the example opposite.

Example: $2\dfrac{1}{2} + 3\dfrac{1}{3} = ?$

Add the whole numbers:

$$2 + 3 = 5$$

Add the fractions:

$$\dfrac{1}{2} + \dfrac{1}{3}$$

Find the common denominator: 6

$$\dfrac{1\ (\times 3)}{2\ (\times 3)} = \dfrac{3}{6}$$

$$\dfrac{1\ (\times 2)}{3\ (\times 2)} = \dfrac{2}{6}$$

Add the fractions:

$$\dfrac{3+2}{6} = \dfrac{5}{6}$$

Add the whole number:

$$5\dfrac{5}{6}$$

Multiplication of fractions

To multiply fractions:

1. Multiply the numerators.
2. Multiply the denominators.
3. Place the product of the numerators over the product of the denominators.
4. Simplify if necessary.

Example: $\dfrac{2}{3} \times \dfrac{5}{7} = ?$

$$\dfrac{2 \times 5}{3 \times 7} = \dfrac{10}{21}$$

To multiply a fraction by a whole number:

1. Multiply only the numerator of the fraction by the whole number.
2. Place the product over the denominator.
3. Simplify if necessary.

Example: $5 \times \dfrac{3}{7} = ?$

$$\dfrac{5}{1} \times \dfrac{3}{7} = \dfrac{5 \times 3}{1 \times 7} = \dfrac{15}{7}$$

Simplify: $\dfrac{15}{7} = 2\dfrac{1}{7}$

To multiply a fraction by a mixed number:

1. Change the mixed number to an improper fraction.
2. Multiply the numerators.
3. Multiply the denominators.
4. Place the product of the numerators over the product of the denominators.
5. Simplify if necessary.

Example: $3\frac{1}{5} \times \frac{3}{4} = ?$

$$3\frac{1}{5} = \frac{16}{5}$$

$$\frac{16}{5} \times \frac{3}{4} = \frac{16 \times 3}{5 \times 4} = \frac{48}{20}$$

Simplify: $\frac{48 \, (\div 4)}{20 \, (\div 4)} = \frac{12}{5} = 2\frac{2}{5}$

Division of fractions

To divide fractions:

1. Invert the terms of the divisor. The divisor is the number that is being divided into the dividend.
2. Use multiplication.
3. Simplify if necessary.

Example: $\frac{1}{3} \div \frac{1}{2} = ?$

$$\underset{\text{dividend}}{\nearrow} \quad \underset{\text{divisor}}{\nwarrow}$$

Invert the divisor: $\frac{1}{2} = \frac{2}{1}$

Multiply: $\frac{1}{3} \times \frac{2}{1} = \frac{1 \times 2}{3 \times 1} = \frac{2}{3}$

To divide a fraction by a whole number:

1. Express the whole number as a fraction.
2. Invert the divisor.
3. Use multiplication.
4. Simplify if necessary.

Example: $\frac{5}{6} \div 2 = ?$

Convert the whole number: $\frac{2}{1}$

Invert: $\frac{2}{1}$ becomes $\frac{1}{2}$

Multiply: $\frac{5}{6} \times \frac{1}{2} = \frac{5 \times 1}{6 \times 2} = \frac{5}{12}$

To divide a fraction by a mixed number:

1. Change the mixed number to an improper fraction.
2. Invert the divisor.
3. Use multiplication.
4. Simplify if necessary.

Example: $\dfrac{3}{4} \div 1\dfrac{1}{8} = ?$

Convert to an improper fraction:

$$1\dfrac{1}{8} = \dfrac{9}{8}$$

Invert the divisor: $\dfrac{9}{8} = \dfrac{8}{9}$

Multiply: $\dfrac{3}{4} \times \dfrac{8}{9} = \dfrac{3 \times 8}{4 \times 9} = \dfrac{24}{36}$

Simplify: $\dfrac{24\,(\div 12)}{36\,(\div 12)} = \dfrac{2}{3}$

▶ DECIMAL NUMBERS

Definitions

Decimal numbers:

- Express the values that describe both whole units and portions of whole units
- Include a decimal point and values to the right and left of the decimal

The numbers written to the left of the decimal point are whole numbers. The numbers written to the right of the decimal point are decimal fractions; that is, fractions with denominators in multiples of 10.

Example: $0.1 = \dfrac{1}{10}$ or one-tenth

$0.01 = \dfrac{1}{100}$ or one-hundredth

$0.001 = \dfrac{1}{1000}$ or one-thousandth

In the number 6.125 there are

6 ones

$\dfrac{1}{10}$ or one-tenth

$\dfrac{2}{100}$ or two-hundredths

$\dfrac{5}{1000}$ or five-thousandths

The size of decimal numbers can be compared by examining the values in each position to the right and left of the decimal point.

> **Example:** Which is larger, 0.5 or 0.05?
>
> 0 ones ⟵—— 0.5 ——⟶ 5 tenths
>
> 0 ones ⟵—— 0.05 ——⟶ 0 tenths, 5 hundredths
>
> Therefore, 0.5 is larger than 0.05.

Rules for Writing Decimal Numbers

1. Always place a zero to the left of the decimal point when there are no whole numbers.

> **Example:** 0.25 not .25

2. Never place a zero to the right of the decimal point.

> **Example:** 1 not 1.0
>
> 1.2 not 1.20

CRITICAL POINT

These rules are extremely important when writing drug dosages. If a drug is ordered as 0.125 mg, the zero placed before the decimal point highlights the point that might otherwise be missed. If 0.125 mg is misread as 125 mg, a fatal drug error could occur. Similarly, a zero placed after the decimal point is unnecessary. A drug order for 6 units is less likely to be misinterpreted than one written as 6.0 units. Missing the decimal point could result in a tenfold error.

Rounding Decimal Numbers

Most calibrated devices used for medication administration are accurate only to the nearest tenth or hundredth. It is acceptable to round dosage calculations to significant digits. As a general rule, if the amount of medication is less than 1 mL, you should round to the nearest hundredth: 1-mL syringes are calibrated to account for this. If the amount of medication is greater than 1 mL, you should round to the nearest tenth.

To round a decimal number:

1. Locate the digit to the right of the one to be retained.
2. If this digit is 5 or greater, add a value of 1 to the numeral to its immediate left.
3. If this digit is less than 5, do not increase the value of the numeral to its immediate left.

Example: Round 1.126 to the nearest hundredth.

The digit in the hundredth position is 2.

The digit to the right is 6.

Increase the value of the numeral in the hundredth place by 1.

The answer is 1.13.

Example: Round 1.13 to the nearest tenth.

The digit in the tenth position is 1.

The digit to the right is 3.

Do not add any value to the tenth.

The answer is 1.1.

Arithmetic of Decimal Numbers

Addition and subtraction of decimal numbers

Decimal points must be lined up vertically, so that, for example, tenths are under tenths and hundredths are under hundredths. It is understood that whole numbers have a decimal point to the right of the ones place.

Example: $1.9 + 0.37 + 2.706 = ?$

$$
\begin{array}{r}
1.9 \\
0.37 \\
+2.706 \\
\hline
4.976
\end{array}
$$

Example: $2.75 - 0.59 = ?$

$$
\begin{array}{r}
2.75 \\
-0.59 \\
\hline
2.16
\end{array}
$$

Example: $4.00 - 3.19 = ?$

$$
\begin{array}{r}
4.00 \\
-3.19 \\
\hline
0.81
\end{array}
$$

Multiplication of decimal numbers

The multiplication of decimal numbers follows the same rules as those for the multiplication of whole numbers, but the placement of the decimal point must be determined separately.

To multiply decimal numbers:

1. Multiply as for whole numbers.
2. Count the number of digits to the right of the decimal point in each of the numbers being multiplied.
3. Add these numbers.
4. Place the decimal point so that this number of digits sits to the right of the decimal point.

Example: $2.162 \times 13.4 = ?$

2.162 has 3 digits to the right of the decimal point.

13.4 has 1 digit to the right of the decimal point.

The answer must have 4 digits to the right of the decimal point.

$$
\begin{array}{r}
2.162 \\
\times\ 13.4 \\
\hline
8648 \\
6486 \\
2162 \\
\hline
289708
\end{array}
$$

Place 4 digits to the right of the decimal point: 28.9708.

Division of decimal numbers

To divide decimal numbers:

1. Write the problem as you would for the division of whole numbers.
2. Move the decimal point to the right of the divisor, so that it becomes a whole number. This is achieved by multiplying by 10, 100, or 1000, and so on.
3. Move the decimal point the same number of positions to the right in the dividend; that is, multiply both the divisor and the dividend by 10, 100, or 1000, and so on.
4. Place a decimal directly above the decimal in the dividend.
5. Divide as for whole numbers.
6. Validate your answer by multiplying the answer by the divisor.

Example: $2.5\overline{)23.75}$

The divisor is 2.5; the dividend is 23.75. Multiply both the divisor and the dividend by 10:

$$2.5 \times 10 = 25$$

$$23.75 \times 10 = 237.5$$

$$
\begin{array}{r}
9.5 \\
25\overline{)237.5} \\
225 \\
\hline
12.5 \\
12.5 \\
\hline
\emptyset
\end{array}
$$

Validation: $9.5 \times 25 = 237.5$

Converting Fractions and Decimal Numbers

To convert a fraction to a decimal, divide the numerator by the denominator.

> Example: $\dfrac{1}{2} = ?$
>
> $1 \div 2 = 0.5$

To convert a decimal number to a fraction:

1. Determine the denominator as 10, 100, or 1000, and so on, by the number of digits to the right of the decimal point.
2. Express as a fraction by placing the number over the selected denominator.
3. Simplify if necessary.

> Example: 0.6 has 1 digit to the right
>
> $= \text{tenths or } \dfrac{6}{10}$
>
> 0.06 has 2 digits to the right
>
> $= \text{hundredths or } \dfrac{6}{100}$
>
> 0.006 has 3 digits to the right
>
> $= \text{thousandths or } \dfrac{6}{1000}$

> Example: 0.06 as a fraction $= ?$
>
> The denominator is 100.
>
> $\dfrac{6}{100} = \dfrac{3}{50}$

To convert a mixed number to a decimal number:

1. Express the mixed number as an improper fraction.
2. Divide the numerator by the denominator.

> Example: $1\dfrac{1}{4} = ?$
>
> $1\dfrac{1}{4} = \dfrac{5}{4} = 1.25$

▶ PERCENTS

Percent means "parts in a hundred"; $\frac{x}{100} = x\%$. Our most frequent encounter with percentages occurs in exam scores. For example, if you answer 90 questions of 100 correctly, then your score is 90%. However, few exams have 100 questions — thankfully! How is percent calculated when there are only 30 rather than 100 parts? The first step is to convert your score to an equivalent fraction. What would your score be if you answered 18 questions of 30 correctly?

Converting Fractions, Decimal Numbers, and Percents

To change a fraction to a percent:

1. Express your score as a fraction.
2. Convert the fraction to a decimal number.
3. Multiply the decimal by 100.
4. Add the percent sign.

Example: You answered 18 questions of 30 correctly.

Express as a fraction: $\dfrac{18}{30}$

Convert: $\dfrac{18}{30} = 0.6$

Multiply: $0.6 \times 100 = 60$

Add sign: 60%

Your score is 60%.

To change a decimal number to a percent:

1. Multiply the decimal by 100.
2. Add the percent sign.

Example: $0.67 = ?$

$0.67 \times 100 = 67$

67%

To change a percent to a fraction:

1. Remove the percent sign.
2. Place the percent number over 100.
3. Simplify if necessary.

> **Example:** $40\% = ?$
>
> 40
>
> $$\frac{40}{100} = \frac{2}{5}$$

To change a percent to a decimal number:

1. Remove the percent sign.
2. Divide by 100.
3. Write the decimal number according to the rules.

> **Example:** $40\% = ?$
>
> 40
>
> $40 \div 100 = .4$
>
> 0.4

▶ POST-TEST

Now that you have reviewed Module 1, check your skills.

Instructions

1. Write the post-test without referring to any resources.

2. Express all fractions in their lowest terms, and change improper fractions to whole numbers and proper fractions.

3. Correct the post-test by using the answer guide starting on page 192. (Value: 1 mark each)

4. If your score is 100%, proceed to Module 2.

5. If your score is less than 100%, review the module topics and rewrite the post-test. If your score is still less than 100%, please seek remedial assistance.

Arithmetic of Whole Numbers

Perform the indicated operations.

1. $\begin{array}{r} 63 \\ +78 \\ \hline \end{array}$
2. $\begin{array}{r} 142 \\ +\ 63 \\ \hline \end{array}$
3. $\begin{array}{r} 741 \\ -121 \\ \hline \end{array}$
4. $\begin{array}{r} 864 \\ -\ 88 \\ \hline \end{array}$

5. $\begin{array}{r} 161 \\ \times\ 11 \\ \hline \end{array}$
6. $\begin{array}{r} 325 \\ \times\ 23 \\ \hline \end{array}$
7. $2125 \div 25 =$
8. $322 \div 14 =$

Fractions

Add the following fractions. Simplify where necessary.

9. $\dfrac{3}{7} + \dfrac{1}{2} =$
10. $\dfrac{1}{3} + \dfrac{7}{8} =$
11. $1\dfrac{1}{2} + \dfrac{1}{6} =$
12. $\dfrac{2}{5} + \dfrac{4}{11} =$

13. $\dfrac{2}{9} + \dfrac{7}{18} =$ 14. $\dfrac{2}{3} + \dfrac{1}{7} =$ 15. $3 + \dfrac{5}{15} =$ 16. $\dfrac{9}{28} + \dfrac{4}{7} =$

Perform the following subtraction of fractions. Simplify where necessary.

17. $\dfrac{1}{3} - \dfrac{1}{4} =$ 18. $\dfrac{5}{7} - \dfrac{2}{3} =$ 19. $2\dfrac{1}{5} - \dfrac{9}{10} =$ 20. $\dfrac{7}{12} - \dfrac{1}{8} =$

21. $18 - \dfrac{3}{5} =$ 22. $\dfrac{5}{6} - \dfrac{1}{4} =$ 23. $\dfrac{4}{5} - \dfrac{1}{2} =$ 24. $\dfrac{1}{2} - \dfrac{1}{3} =$

Multiply the following fractions. Simplify where necessary.

25. $\dfrac{2}{7} \times \dfrac{1}{2} =$ 26. $\dfrac{3}{4} \times \dfrac{1}{6} =$ 27. $1\dfrac{1}{8} \times \dfrac{3}{4} =$ 28. $\dfrac{3}{7} \times 9 =$

29. $\dfrac{2}{5} \times \dfrac{3}{5} =$ 30. $16 \times \dfrac{1}{16} =$ 31. $5\dfrac{1}{3} \times \dfrac{1}{3} =$ 32. $\dfrac{4}{11} \times \dfrac{1}{2} =$

Perform the following division of fractions. Simplify where necessary.

33. $\dfrac{3}{5} \div \dfrac{1}{4} =$ 34. $\dfrac{7}{9} \div \dfrac{2}{3} =$ 35. $2 \div \dfrac{5}{6} =$ 36. $\dfrac{1}{2} \div \dfrac{3}{4} =$

37. $\dfrac{5}{9} \div \dfrac{1}{3} =$ 38. $\dfrac{3}{7} \div \dfrac{2}{3} =$ 39. $1\dfrac{3}{5} \div \dfrac{3}{4} =$ 40. $2\dfrac{3}{8} \div 1\dfrac{1}{4} =$

Express the following as improper fractions.

41. $3\dfrac{12}{27} =$ 42. $9\dfrac{3}{8} =$

Change these improper fractions to mixed or whole numbers.

43. $\dfrac{18}{5} =$ 44. $\dfrac{19}{7} =$ 45. $\dfrac{44}{11} =$ 46. $\dfrac{260}{9} =$

47. $\dfrac{28}{6} =$ 48. $\dfrac{16}{10} =$

Find the lowest common denominator.

49. $\dfrac{6}{10}$ and $\dfrac{2}{6}$ 50. $\dfrac{4}{9}$ and $\dfrac{3}{4}$ 51. $\dfrac{2}{7}$ and $\dfrac{21}{77}$ 52. $\dfrac{2}{5}$ and $\dfrac{2}{3}$

Reduce each expression to lowest terms.

53. $\dfrac{45}{108} =$ 54. $\dfrac{24}{96} =$ 55. $\dfrac{9}{3} =$ 56. $\dfrac{13}{52} =$

57. Which of the following is a proper fraction?

$$1\frac{1}{14} \quad \text{or} \quad \frac{7}{5} \quad \text{or} \quad \frac{1}{2}$$

58. Which of the following is a mixed number?

$$1\frac{2}{3} \quad \text{or} \quad \frac{2}{2} \quad \text{or} \quad \frac{15}{7}$$

59. Which of the following is an improper fraction?

$$1\frac{2}{7} \quad \text{or} \quad \frac{9}{8} \quad \text{or} \quad \frac{161}{162}$$

Find the following equivalent fractions.

60. $\dfrac{9}{42} = \dfrac{3}{?}$ 61. $\dfrac{6}{14} = \dfrac{?}{42}$ 62. $\dfrac{13}{78} = \dfrac{?}{12}$

63. $\dfrac{5}{16} = \dfrac{25}{?}$ 64. $\dfrac{33}{36} = \dfrac{11}{?}$

Decimal Numbers

Add the following decimal numbers. Round to the nearest hundredth.

65. $1.33 + 2.5 =$ 66. $4.2 + 6.11 =$ 67. $81.7 + 0.324 =$

68. $1.487 + 6.9 + 2 =$

Perform the following subtraction of decimal numbers. Round each answer to the nearest tenth.

69. $7.8 - 3.3 =$ 70. $9.2 - 6.521 =$ 71. $2.9 - 1.6001 =$

72. $18.9 - 16.42 =$

Multiply the following decimal numbers.

73. $4.6 \times 0.3 =$ 74. $6.8 \times 3.3 =$ 75. $5.1 \times 5.6 =$

76. $7.4 \times 1.6 =$

Perform the following division of decimal numbers.

77. $5.4 \div 2.7 =$ 78. $13.86 \div 2.2 =$ 79. $12.3 \div 2.5 =$

80. $15 \div 2.5 =$

Round the following numbers to the nearest tenth.

81. 6.23   82. 81.73   83. 7.46   84. 7.88

Round the following numbers to the nearest hundredth.

85. 2.915   86. 3.452   87. 6.426   88. 182.614

Percents

Complete the following table using the given information. Follow the example provided in the first line of the table. Express fractions in their lowest terms.

Fraction	Decimal Number	Percent
$\frac{2}{3}$	0.67	67%
(89)	0.22	(90)
(91)	(92)	52%
$\frac{1}{5}$	(93)	(94)
(95)	0.6	(96)
(97)	2.3	(98)
$1\frac{1}{8}$	(99)	(100)

Your Score:	/100	=	%

Did you achieve 100%?

YES — Proceed to Module 2.

NO — Analyze your areas of weakness and review this module; then rewrite the post-test. If your score is still less than 100%, please seek remedial assistance.

Ratio and Proportion

▶ MODULE TOPICS

- Ratio
  - Definition
  - Expressing ratios as fractions, decimal numbers, and percents
- Proportion
  - Definition
  - Using proportion for dosage calculation
  - Alternative solution

▶ INTRODUCTION

This module provides the foundation concepts for dosage calculation. The module provides a review of the terms *ratio* and *proportion* and the expression of ratios as fractions, decimal numbers, and percents. Although you will certainly be familiar with these concepts and terms, you may not have applied them recently; thus, the review will be helpful.

▶ RATIO

Definition

A ratio is a relationship that exists between two quantities. *Ratio* is a way of expressing a part of a whole. For example, 1:5 means 1 in 5 parts.

It is very important to be certain you are choosing the correct numbers for a ratio equation.

> **Example:** Out of a basket of 200 apples, 57 are red and the remaining ones are green. The ratio of red apples in the basket is 57:200 (read "57 to 200"). The ratio of green apples in the basket is 143:200. The ratio of red apples to green apples is 57:143.

Ratios are frequently used in drug calculations. The strength of a medication can be expressed as a ratio.

> **Example:** A drug solution contains 1:500; that is, 1 part drug in 500 parts of solution.

▶ EXERCISE 2.1

Complete the following exercise without referring to the above text. Correct your answers by using the answer guide starting on page 192. (Value: 1 mark each)

1. You answered 18 questions correctly on an exam with 20 questions. What is the ratio of incorrect to correct answers?

2. For the exam results in question 1, what is the ratio of correct to total answers?

3. A drug label states, "1:1000." The drug is in solution. Write out the meaning of this ratio.

4. A bottle of liquid medication states that each teaspoon contains 25 units. Express the ratio of units per teaspoon.

5. In every hour of television programming that you watch, you also "enjoy" 12 minutes of advertising. Express the following as a ratio: time of advertising (in minutes) to time of actual program (in minutes).

Your Score:	/5	=	%

Expressing Ratios as Fractions, Decimal Numbers, and Percents

A ratio may be expressed as a fraction, a decimal number, or a percent.

To convert a ratio to a fraction:

1. Place the first digit in the ratio over the second digit.
2. Simplify the fraction.

> **Example:** 2:50 as a fraction
>
> $$\frac{2}{50}$$
>
> Lowest term: $\dfrac{1}{25}$

To convert a ratio to a decimal number:

1. Express the ratio as a fraction.
2. Divide the numerator into the denominator.
3. Follow the rules for writing decimals.

> **Example:** 1:10 as a decimal
>
> Express as a fraction: $\dfrac{1}{10}$
>
> Divide: 1 divided by 10 is .1
>
> Apply rules: 0.1

To convert a ratio to a percent:

1. Express the ratio as a fraction.
2. Convert the fraction to a decimal number (divide the numerator by the denominator).
3. Multiply the decimal number by 100.
4. Add the percent sign.

> **Example:** 1:20 as a percent
>
> $$\frac{1}{20} = 0.05$$
>
> $0.05 \times 100 = 5$
>
> 5%

To convert a percent to a ratio:

1. Place the percent over 100.
2. Simplify the fraction.
3. Express as a ratio.

Example: $50\% = \dfrac{50}{100} = \dfrac{5}{10} = \dfrac{1}{2} = 1:2$

$0.5\% = \dfrac{0.5}{100} = \dfrac{5}{1000} = \dfrac{1}{200} = 1:200$

▶ **EXERCISE 2.2**

Convert ratios, fractions, decimal numbers, and percents. Complete the table without referring to the above text. Express fractions in lowest terms. Correct your answers by using the answer guide starting on page 192. (Value: 1 mark each)

Ratio	Fraction	Decimal Number	Percent
2:50	(1)	(2)	(3)
(4)	$\dfrac{1}{10}$	(5)	(6)
(7)	(8)	0.78	(9)
(10)	(11)	(12)	49%
(13)	$\dfrac{50}{1}$	(14)	(15)

Your Score:	/15 =	%

▶ **PROPORTION**

Definition

Proportion is the expression of two equivalent ratios. The two ratios are separated by an equal sign. The proportion 2:3 = 4:6 is read "two is to three as four is to six." In a true proportion, the product of the means equals the product of the extremes.

Example: 2:3 = 4:6

means

2:3 = 4:6

extremes

$2 \times 6 = 3 \times 4$

$12 = 12$

Multiply the extremes and place the product to the left of the equal sign. Multiply the means and place the product to the right of the equal sign.

Example: $10:2 = 5:1$

$10 =$

$10:2 = 5:1$

$10 = 10$

Using Proportion for Dosage Calculation

A proportion equation can be used to solve for an unknown quantity. The proportion equation is the simplest and most accurate approach to calculating drug dosages. In these situations, you have a known ratio; for example, the drug label states 325 mg per tablet or a ratio of 325:1. Another label states 100 mg in 2 mL or 100 mg:2 mL. The dosage that you wish to give is the unknown ratio. You know what strength to give, but you must determine the volume to give (the number of tablets or millilitres, for example).

To solve for an unknown value (x) using proportion:

1. Write the known ratio first.
2. Write the unknown ratio.
3. Set up the proportion.
4. Multiply the extremes and the means; place the unknown value on the left.
5. Solve for the unknown. Recall that you must divide both sides of an equation by the same number.
6. Validate your answer. Substitute the answer for x in the equation. Multiply the extremes and the means. The numbers should be the same on both sides of the equal sign.

Example: $200:4 - 50:x$

$200 \times x = 4 \times 50$

$200x = 200$

$\dfrac{200x}{200} = \dfrac{200}{200}$

$x = 1$

Validation: $200:4 = 50:1$

$200 \times 1 = 4 \times 50$

$200 = 200$

NOTE: The *means* are the values in the middle; the *extremes* are the values on the ends.

Alternative Solution

You may be more familiar with writing a proportion as two fractions and using cross multiplication.

To solve for an unknown value (x) using fractions as proportion:

1. Write the known ratio as a fraction.

2. Write the unknown ratio as a fraction using x for the unknown value.

3. Determine the cross multiplication: multiply the numerator of each fraction by the denominator of the other fraction.

4. Solve for x. Divide both sides of the equation by the same value.

5. Validate your answer by substituting the value of x into the original equation.

Example: $5:10 = 7:x$

$$\frac{5}{10} = \frac{7}{x} \qquad \frac{5}{10} \diagdown \frac{7}{x}$$

$$5x = 70$$

$$\frac{5x}{5} = \frac{70}{5}$$

$$x = 14$$

Validation: $5:10 = 7:14$

$$\frac{5}{10} = \frac{7}{14}$$

$$70 = 70$$

CRITICAL POINT

To ensure accuracy, you are advised to solve for x using one method and to validate your answer using the other method.

▶ EXERCISE 2.3

Complete the following exercise without referring to the above text. Express answers in whole or decimal numbers. Round to the nearest hundredth. Correct your answers by using the answer guide starting on page 192. (Questions 1 to 15, value: 1 mark each)

Solve for x.

1. $2:3 = x:12$

2. $1:5 = x:125$

3. $5:7 = 15:x$

4. $25:1 = 50:x$

5. $10:1 = 15:x$

6. $75:6 = 50:x$

7. $35:x = 100:1$

8. $0.25:1 = 0.125:x$

9. $250:1000 = x:1$

10. $10:1000 = x:100$

11. $1:8 = \frac{1}{2}:x$

12. $18:x = 5:300$

13. $0.5:2 = x:4$

14. $\frac{1}{4}:x = 6:12$

15. $x:6 = \frac{1}{100}:\frac{1}{10}$

For each of the following problems, show your work and validate the answer (show the proof). (Value: 2 marks each; 1 for a correct answer, 1 for validation)

16. To make 6 cups of coffee, you use 4 scoops of ground coffee beans. How many scoops do you need to use to make 24 cups of coffee?

17. A pancake recipe requires 1 cup of milk and $1\frac{1}{2}$ cups of mix. You have 6 cups of mix. How much milk should you add?

18. You are making party bags for birthday party guests and you want to put in 1 package of gum with 3 packages of mints. How many packages of gum do you need for 45 packages of mints?

19. At the last hot dog day, 22 children ate 33 hot dogs. How many hot dogs would you prepare for a class of 28 children?

20. The fruit drink recipe calls for 1 cup of lime juice to 3 cups of apple juice. How much lime juice would you add to 24 cups of apple juice?

Your Score: /25 = %

▶ EXERCISE 2.4

Complete the following exercise without referring to the above text. Correct your answers by using the answer guide starting on page 192. (Value: 1 mark each)

1. Define the term *ratio*.

2. Define the term *proportion*.

For the following situation, answer questions 3 to 5.

A plane has 350 passengers and 10 crew members. Sixty-five percent of the total group are male.

3. What is the ratio of males to females?

4. What is the ratio of males to the total group?

5. What is the ratio of crew members to passengers?

For questions 6 to 10, solve for x.

6. $5:x = 7:35$

7. $9:x = 10:100$

8. $3.5:x = 4.5:9$

9. $\dfrac{x}{100} = \dfrac{5}{20}$

10. $\dfrac{8}{x} = \dfrac{12}{6}$

11. Express $\dfrac{1}{10}$ as a decimal number.

12. Express 1.23 as a percent.

13. Convert 33.5% to a decimal number.

14. Express 45:90 as a fraction; reduce to lowest terms.

15. In this proportion, state the means and the extremes: 2:3 = 4:6.

Your Score:	/15	=	%

▶ POST-TEST

Instructions

1. Write the post-test without referring to any resources.

2. Correct the post-test by using the answer guide starting on page 192. (Value: 1 mark each)

Solve for x. Express answers as whole or decimal numbers.

1. $3:x = 1:15$

2. $9:x = 3:4$

3. $\dfrac{x}{100} = \dfrac{5}{20}$

4. $\dfrac{25}{1} = \dfrac{100}{x}$

5. $\dfrac{8}{x} = \dfrac{12}{6}$

6. $\dfrac{1}{50} = \dfrac{x}{150}$

Express the following ratios as fractions, decimal numbers, and percents. Reduce fractions to lowest terms. (Value: 1 mark each)

Ratio	Fraction	Decimal Number	Percent
1:100	(7)	(8)	(9)
1:5	(10)	(11)	(12)
4:1000	(13)	(14)	(15)

Solve for x. (Value: 1 mark each)

16. $\dfrac{0.25}{1} = \dfrac{0.125}{x}$

17. $\dfrac{2.2}{1} = \dfrac{x}{75}$

18. $\dfrac{1000}{1.5} = \dfrac{x}{3}$

19. $60:5 = 150:x$

20. You buy 7 oranges and 5 apples. What is the ratio of oranges to apples?

21. There are 40 patients and 8 staff members. What is the ratio of patients to staff? Express as a ratio in lowest terms.

22. Your score is 85% on a math exam. What is the ratio of correct to incorrect answers? Express as a ratio in lowest terms.

23. Your coffeemaker instructions state that 6 scoops of ground coffee make 8 cups of coffee. How many scoops are needed to make 2 cups?

24. Define the term *ratio*.

25. Define the term *proportion*.

For each problem, write the proportion equation and solve for *x*.

26. There are 2 baskets of fruit with equal ratios of oranges and apples. Basket 1 has 3 oranges and 5 apples. Basket 2 has 9 oranges. How many apples are there in Basket 2?

27. Two classes of children are going on a field trip, and you want the same ratio of children from grades 2 and 3 in each bus. The first bus has 8 grade 2 students and 12 grade 3 students. The second bus has 10 grade 2 students. How many grade 3 students should there be in the second bus?

28. A basketball player has a scoring average of 18 of 25 shots. How many baskets will she likely score if she takes 50 shots?

29. The recipe calls for 1 cup of milk and 2 cups of flour. How much milk should be used for 3 cups of flour?

30. A necklace has 5 blue beads to 12 red beads. How many blue beads should there be for 48 red beads?

Your Score: /30 = %

Did you achieve 100%?

YES — Proceed to Module 3.

NO — Analyze your areas of weakness and review this module; then rewrite the post-test. If your score is still less than 100%, please seek remedial assistance.

Systems of Measurement

▶ **MODULE TOPICS**

- Systems of measurement
  - Household system
  - Apothecary system
  - SI system
- Rules for writing SI symbols
- Converting SI subunits to base units
- Common conversions among systems
- Twenty-four-hour time

▶ **INTRODUCTION**

This module reviews three systems of measurement: the household system, which you will easily recognize, the apothecary system, and the SI system, which some refer to as the *metric system*. Drugs, for the most part, are measured in milligrams and may be dissolved in millilitres of a liquid; this module lays the foundation for understanding the medication order. Learn the content in the module and seek out opportunities to use the information. For example, ask your instructor to provide syringes (measured in millilitres) and calibrated devices such as plastic containers measured in ounces. Using the equipment, measure and compare the volumes.

Module 3 also teaches you to convert from one unit to another, for example, milligrams to grams. Again, this is important to know when calculating drug doses because the order may appear in one unit and the drug supply may be measured in another.

▶ **SYSTEMS OF MEASUREMENT**

Three major systems of measurement have been used to calculate drug doses: the household system, the apothecary system, and the SI system.

Although it is not common to do conversions from one system of measurement to another, there are a few instances in which this occurs, particularly in home settings or in instructions to a patient and family regarding over-the-counter (OTC) drugs.

CRITICAL POINT

If you are unfamiliar with any drug order written in nonstandardized units, consult with the prescribing physician or a pharmacist.

Household System

The household system uses measures such as *teaspoons* and *tablespoons*. These measures do not provide accuracy but may be used for medications taken in the home. Common household measures include the following:

- teaspoon (tsp.)
- tablespoon (tbsp.)
- pint (pt.)
- quart (qt.)
- gallon (gal.)

Apothecary System

The apothecary system is a very old one whose basic units include *minims, ounces,* and *grains.* These measures have almost become obsolete, except for some drug orders for laxatives, antacids, and cough syrups that are written in ounces.[1] It's useful for you to be familiar with some of the units of this system, since patients and families might be accustomed to these measures.[2] See Appendix A for approximate equivalents among the systems of measurement.

SI System

The SI system, or *Système international d'unités,* is essentially an expanded version of the metric system. It is a decimal system based on the number 10. The SI system has been widely adopted throughout the world — by 98% of the world's population.

There are seven base units or building blocks in this system. The *base units* you will encounter most often in relation to medications are outlined in Table 3.1.

TABLE 3.1 Common Base Units

Unit	Quantity Measured	Symbol
metre[3]	length	m
kilogram[4]	weight	kg
mole	substance	mol

You are probably familiar with *metre* and *kilogram.* You have no doubt bought a metre of fabric or driven 100 km. A metre is approximately the distance between the bottom of a door and its doorknob. Possibly you have bought a kilogram of meat. A kilogram is approximately equal in weight to a one-litre carton of milk.

Mole is possibly not familiar to you. It isn't a measurement of weight. A mole is an amount of substance, defined as the number of atoms in exactly 12 g of the carbon-12

---

[1] Some aspirin products are still labelled in grains.
[2] *Pounds* and *inches* are also part of this system.
[3] The spellings *meter* and *metre* are both correct. The former is commonly used in the United States; the latter is used by most other nations.
[4] The unit of weight in the SI system is *kilogram*; the unit of weight in the metric system is *gram.*

isotope. The number of atoms in a mole of a substance is 6.02×10^{23}. If your curiosity is aroused by this definition, you might appreciate a further explanation. An anonymous and creative author described one mole of peas as follows: "10^{23} average-size peas would cover 250 planets the size of Earth with a blanket of peas 1 metre deep!" Obviously, one mole of peas occupies a much larger volume than does one mole of the electrolyte potassium chloride.

Many chemistry reports are expressed in molar units. This will become more significant to you when you read drug plasma levels reported in moles.

Examples:	
insulin:	30–170 pmol/L (picomoles per litre)
digoxin:	< 2.6 nmol/L (nanomoles per litre)
lithium:	0.6–1.2 mmol/L (millimoles per litre)

NOTE: Laboratory values can vary slightly. Check the normal values written on the lab reports in your particular clinical setting.

In addition to these base units, one other measurement is not an official SI unit but is of interest to health professionals. This is the unit of volume called the *litre*. It is used for example, for intravenous fluids, which are packaged in one-litre (1000 mL) containers.

Because the metre, kilogram, mole, and litre are relatively large units, the SI system uses prefixes to denote multiple units and subunits. There are 16 prefixes; those used most frequently in relation to drug therapy are listed in Table 3.2. These numerical values are important when converting base units and subunits of the SI system. You will do this frequently when administering medications and intravenous fluids to your patients. Mastering this module is an important step toward competence in calculating dosages.

TABLE 3.2 SI Subunits

Prefix	Symbol	Numerical Value
kilo	k	1000
hecto	h	100
deca[5]	dk	10
deci	d	0.1
centi	c	0.01
milli	m	0.001
micro	µ or mc	0.000 001
nano	n	0.000 000 001

NOTE: The official symbol for *micro* is µ; however, some references use *mc*. Both abbreviations are acceptable; *mc* is used throughout this book.

---

[5] Some sources use *deka* for the prefix and *da* for the symbol.

▶ EXERCISE 3.1

Review Table 3.2. Complete the following exercise without referring to the above text. Correct your answers by using the answer guide starting on page 192. (Value: 1 mark each unless otherwise indicated)

Give the SI symbol for each of the following prefixes:

1. kilo
2. deci
3. centi
4. milli
5. micro

Write out the numerical value for each of the following prefixes:

6. kilo
7. nano
8. deca
9. milli
10. micro
11. centi
12. hecto
13. Name the eight subunits outlined in Table 3.2, from largest to smallest. (Value: 8 marks)

Your Score:	/20	=	%

▶ RULES FOR WRITING SI SYMBOLS

1. Symbols of units are written in lowercase initials, except when they are named after a person.

> **Examples:** degree Celsius = °C
>
> metre = m

2. Symbols are not pluralized. They are written without a period, except when the symbol occurs at the end of a sentence. It is correct to pluralize the metric unit name; thus, *25 kilograms* is correct.

> **Examples:** He weighs 10 kg.
>
> Ten kilograms is correct.

3. A space must separate the digits from the symbols.

> **Example:** 1 mL not 1mL

4. Decimals should be used instead of fractions.

> **Example:** 0.5 mg not $\frac{1}{2}$ mg

5. A zero should always be placed before the decimal point when there is no whole number.

> **Example:** 0.5 not .5

6. To avoid confusion with the number *1*, the word *litre* should be written in full or a capital *L* should be used. The capital *L* is also used with prefixes.

NOTE: The capital *L* is preferred in Canada, Australia, and the United States.

> **Examples:** litre = L
>
> millilitre = mL

7. Writing numbers with more than three digits — that is, in the thousands — is slightly different from the traditional method. No comma is used. Instead, a space is left, as shown in the examples

> **Examples:** 23 000
>
> 217 860

opposite. For the number 1000, it is optional to leave a space; thus, both 1000 and 1 000 are correct.

NOTE: The Metric Commission of Canada states that spaces are used to separate long numbers into three-digit blocks. With four-digit numbers, the space is optional.

8. Although *cc, cubic centimetre*, isn't a standard SI unit, it may be used by health professionals — one cubic centimetre is approximately equal to one millilitre.

▶ EXERCISE 3.2

Complete the following exercise without referring to the above text. Correct your answers by using the answer guide starting on page 192. (Value: 1 mark each)

Indicate which of the following correctly adhere to the rules for writing SI symbols. Circle your choices.

1. metre = m or M
2. 10 kilograms = 10 kg or 10 kgs
3. $\frac{1}{2}$ millilitre = $\frac{1}{2}$ mL or 0.5 mL
4. litre = L or l
5. One thousand millilitres = 1000 mL or 1000 ml
6. One-half litre = .5 L or 0.5 L or 0.5 l
7. One thousand and fifty milligrams = 1050 mgms or 1050 mg
8. millilitre = mL or ml
9. Write fifty-one thousand, five hundred seventeen according to the SI rules.
10. True or false? One cubic centimetre is approximately equal to one millilitre.

Your Score:	/10 =	%

▶ CONVERTING SI SUBUNITS TO BASE UNITS

The most common subunits encountered in drug therapy are *milli* and *micro*. In addition, you will frequently encounter *centi* in measurements of height or length. Table 3.3 illustrates some relationships involving units of the SI system.

TABLE 3.3 Units and Values

Unit	Value
gram (g) to milligram (mg)	1 g = 1000 mg
gram (g) to microgram (mcg)	1 g = 1 000 000 mcg
milligram (mg) to microgram (mcg)	1 mg = 1000 mcg
litre (L) to millilitre (mL)	1 L = 1000 mL
metre (m) to centimetre (cm)	1 m = 100 cm
metre (m) to millimetre (mm)	1 m = 1000 mm

Conversion of subunits to base units and vice versa is a simple exercise involving multiplication or division by 10, 100, or 1000. The trick, of course, is to remember whether to multiply or divide! The simplest approach is to use a proportion equation.

Method A: extremes = means
Method B: cross multiplication

Problem: Convert 10 g to milligrams.

Method A: Extremes = Means

Known ratio: 1 g = 1000 mg

Unknown ratio: 10 g = x mg

1 g:1000 mg = 10 g:x mg

$1x = 1000 \times 10$

$x = 10\ 000$

10 g = 10 000 mg

Validation: $\dfrac{1\ g}{1000\ mg} = \dfrac{10\ g}{x\ mg}$

$1x = 1000 \times 10$

$x = 10\ 000$ mg

Method B: Cross Multiplication

Known ratio: $\dfrac{1 \text{ g}}{1000 \text{ mg}}$

Unknown ratio: $\dfrac{10 \text{ g}}{x \text{ mg}}$

$$\frac{1 \text{ g}}{1000 \text{ mg}} = \frac{10 \text{ g}}{x \text{ mg}}$$

$$1x = 1000 \times 10$$

$$x = 10\ 000$$

$$10 \text{ g} = 10\ 000 \text{ mg}$$

Validation: 1 g:1000 mg = 10 g:10 000 mg

$$1 \times 10\ 000 = 1000 \times 10$$

$$10\ 000 = 10\ 000$$

CRITICAL POINT

If you use the extremes = means method to solve, validate your answer by substituting the answer for x in the equation and using cross multiplication. If you use cross multiplication, validate your answer by inserting the answer for x and performing the extremes = means method.

Remember to write the proportion with the known ratio on the left and the unknown ratio on the right. Be sure that each side of the equation is set up in the same way. In the previous example, the known ratio is stated as grams:milligrams, so the unknown ratio must also be stated as grams:milligrams. Examine the following problem and determine the various ways that the proportion could be stated.

Problem: How many milligrams are there in 0.2 g?

There are at least three ways to state a proportion equation to solve this question. In each proportion, the relationship is the same for both sides of the equation.

Solution 1: 1 g:1000 mg = 0.2 g:x mg
Solution 2: 1 g:0.2 g = 1000 mg:x mg
Solution 3: 1000 mg:1 g = x mg:0.2 g

Solutions for each equation show that the proportion equations all yield the same answer.

Method A: Extremes = Means

Solution 1: $1\,g:1000\,mg = 0.2\,g:x\,mg$

$1x = 1000 \times 0.2$

$x = 200$

Answer is 200 mg.

Validation: $\dfrac{1\,g}{1000\,mg} = \dfrac{0.2\,g}{200\,mg}$

$1 \times 200 = 1000 \times 0.2$

$200 = 200$

Solution 2: $1\,g:0.2\,g = 1000\,mg:x\,mg$

$1x = 0.2 \times 1000$

$x = 200$

Answer is 200 mg.

Validation: $\dfrac{1\,g}{0.2\,g} = \dfrac{1000\,mg}{200\,mg}$

$1 \times 200 = 0.2 \times 1000$

$200 = 200$

Solution 3: $1000\,mg:1\,g = x\,mg:0.2\,g$

$1x = 1000 \times 0.2$

$x = 200$

Answer is 200 mg.

Validation: $\dfrac{1000\,mg}{1\,g} = \dfrac{200\,mg}{0.2\,g}$

$1000 \times 0.2 = 1 \times 200$

$200 = 200$

Method B: Cross Multiplication

Solution 1: $$\frac{1\text{ g}}{1000\text{ mg}} = \frac{0.2\text{ g}}{x\text{ mg}}$$

$1x = 1000 \times 0.2$

$x = 200$

Answer is 200 mg.

Validation: 1 g:1000 mg = 0.2 g:200 mg

$1 \times 200 = 1000 \times 0.2$

$200 = 200$

Solution 2: $$\frac{1\text{ g}}{0.2\text{ g}} = \frac{1000\text{ mg}}{x\text{ mg}}$$

$1x = 0.2 \times 1000$

$x = 200$

Answer is 200 mg.

Validation: 1 g:0.2 g = 1000 mg:200 mg

$1 \times 200 = 0.2 \times 1000$

$200 = 200$

Solution 3: $$\frac{1000\text{ mg}}{1\text{ g}} = \frac{x\text{ mg}}{0.2\text{ g}}$$

$1x = 1000 \times 0.2$

$x = 200$

Answer is 200 mg.

Validation: 1000 mg:1 g = 200 mg:0.2 g

$1000 \times 0.2 = 1 \times 200$

$200 = 200$

▶ EXERCISE 3.3

Complete the following exercise without referring to the above text. Correct your answers by using the answer guide starting on page 192. (Value: 1 mark each)

1. 1 L = _____ mL
2. 1 kg = _____ g
3. 1 m = _____ cm
4. 1 cc = _____ mL
5. 1 g = _____ mcg
6. 250 mL = _____ L
7. 0.5 L = _____ mL
8. 2 m = _____ cm
9. 1 mg = _____ mcg
10. 1000 mcg = _____ g

Your Score: /10   =   %

▶ COMMON CONVERSIONS AMONG SYSTEMS

Because of the common usage of *inches, pounds,* and *fluid ounces* by the public and by professionals, it is practical to know the following conversions from the SI system to the household and apothecary systems. Table 3.4 lists these common conversions.

TABLE 3.4 Common Conversions

Quantity Measured	SI Units	Household/ Apothecary Units	Relationship
weight	kg	pound (lb.)	1 kg = 2.2 lb.
height	cm	inch (in.)	2.54 cm = 1 in.
		foot (ft.)	30.48 cm = 1 ft. (12 in.)
volume	mL	teaspoon (tsp.)	5 mL = 1 tsp.
		tablespoon (tbsp.)	15 mL = 1 tbsp.
		fluid ounces (fl. oz.)	30 mL = 1 fl. oz.
		cup (c.)	240 mL ≅ 1 c.
		quart (qt.)	1000 mL[6] = 1 qt.

---

[6] An imperial quart is 1136 mL and a U.S. quart is 946 mL.

Example: 2 kg = x lb.

  1 kg:2.2 lb. = 2 kg:x lb.

  $1x = 2.2 \times 2$

  $x = 4.4$

Answer is 4.4 lb.

Example: 88 lb. = x kg

  1 kg:2.2 lb. = x kg:88 lb.

  $2.2x = 88$

  $x = (88 \div 2.2) = 40$

Answer is 40 kg.

Example: 3 fl. oz. = x mL

  1 fl. oz.:30 mL = 3 fl. oz.:x mL

  $1x = 30 \times 3$

  $x = 90$

Answer is 90 mL.

▶ EXERCISE 3.4

Review Table 3.4 and master the conversions before completing the following exercise. Answer the questions without referring to resources. Correct your answers by using the answer guide starting on page 192. (Value: 1 mark each)

You are admitting Mr. Jones, who cannot be weighed. He tells you that his weight is 175 lb.

  1. Convert Mr. Jones's weight to kilograms.
  2. Round to the nearest tenth.
  3. Round to the nearest kilogram.

Tim's height is 140 cm.

  4. Express Tim's height in inches. Round to the nearest whole number.
  5. Express Tim's height in feet and inches.
  6. A label reads, "For ages 2 to 3, give 1 tsp." Convert this measurement to millilitres.
  7. An order is Magnolax 1 fl. oz. Convert to millilitres.
  8. Jane's height is 5 feet 3 inches; express her height in centimetres. Round to the nearest whole number.
  9. A label reads, "10 mL for ages 10 to 12." Convert this measurement to teaspoons.
  10. A bottle contains 5 fl. oz. Convert this to millilitres.

Convert. Round to the nearest tenth.

  11. 27 kg = _____ lb.
  12. 3 tsp. = _____ mL

13. 30 in. = _____ cm
14. 4.3 kg = _____ lb.
15. 5 ft. 6 in. = _____ cm
16. 2 fl. oz. = _____ mL
17. 149 lb. = _____ kg
18. 1 c. = _____ mL
19. 154 cm = _____ in.
20. 240 mL = _____ fl. oz.

Your Score: _____ /20 = _____ %

▶ TWENTY-FOUR-HOUR TIME

To encourage precision in documentation and to prevent medication administration errors, most care settings use the 24-hour clock. If you are not accustomed to expressing time in this way, review the following explanation.

With 24-hour time, the time is expressed as four digits. Midnight is point zero. The first two digits express the number of hours since midnight; thus, 0100 is one hour after midnight, whereas 1300 is thirteen hours after midnight. The latter would be commonly expressed as 1 P.M. The second two digits express the number of minutes in that hour; thus, 0120 refers to twenty minutes past 1 A.M. Figure 3.1 illustrates the 24-hour clock.

To convert hours after 12 noon, add 12 to the time. Therefore, 6 P.M. is 6 + 12 = 1800.

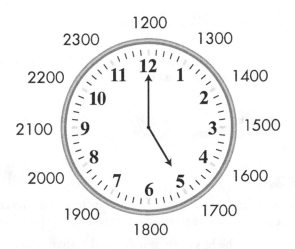

FIGURE 3.1 The 24-hour clock. Explanation: 1 P.M. = 1300 h; 2 P.M. = 1400 h; 3 P.M. = 1500 h; 4 P.M. = 1600 h; 5 P.M. = 1700 h; 6 P.M. = 1800 h; 7 P.M. = 1900 h; 8 P.M. = 2000 h; 9 P.M. = 2100 h; 10 P.M. = 2200 h; 11 P.M. = 2300 h; 12 P.M. = 1200 h.

▶ EXERCISE 3.5

Complete the following exercise without referring to the above text. Correct your answers using the answer guide starting on page 192. (Value: 1 mark each)

Convert the following times to 24-hour time.

1. 1:15 P.M.
2. 6:45 A.M.
3. 9:20 A.M.
4. 8 P.M.
5. 9:08 P.M.
6. 11:23 P.M.
7. 10:19 P.M.
8. 2:10 A.M.

Convert the following 24-hour times to conventional time (the 12-hour clock).

9. 1557 h
10. 2130 h
11. 1415 h
12. 2359 h
13. 0005 h
14. 0300 h
15. 2230 h
16. 1100 h
17. 1950 h
18. 1705 h
19. The chart indicates that the next dose of medication should be given at 1416 h. What time is this on a 12-hour clock?
20. You must start an intravenous infusion at 2:30 P.M. Your workplace uses 24-hour time. What time will you record on the chart?

Your Score:	/20	=	%

▶ EXERCISE 3.6

Complete the following exercise without referring to the above text. Correct your answers by using the answer guide starting on page 192. (Value: 1 mark each)

1. Complete the sentence: The SI system is a decimal system that is based on the number _____.
2. In the SI system, what is the name for the base unit of length?
3. In the SI system, what is the name for the base unit of mass?
4. In the SI system, what is the name for the base unit of substance?

Complete the table by inserting the symbol for the prefix.

Prefix	Symbol
(5) kilo	
(6) hecto	
(7) deca	
(8) deci	
(9) centi	
(10) milli	
(11) micro	
(12) nano	

13. State the conversion for kilograms to pounds.

14. How many millilitres are in a teaspoon?

15. How many centimetres are in one inch?

Your Score:	/15	=	%

▶ **POST-TEST**

Instructions

1. Write the post-test without referring to any resources.

2. Correct the post-test by using the answer guide starting on page 192. (Value: 1 mark each)

Convert each of the following measurements.

1. 10 g = _____ mg   2. 50 mg = _____ g   3. 0.25 g = _____ mg

4. 1.25 mg = _____ mcg   5. 1 L = _____ mL   6. 2 kg = _____ g

7. 350 mg = _____ g   8. 1.5 m = _____ cm   9. 0.7 g = _____ mcg

Convert the following household measurements to SI units. Round to the nearest whole number.

10. 3.4 fl. oz. = _____ mL   11. 2 tsp. = _____ mL   12. 35 kg = _____ lbs.

13. 143 lb. = _____ kg   14. 26 in. = _____ cm   15. 42 cm = _____ in.

16. 32 fl. oz. = _____ mL   17. 72 fl. oz. = _____ mL

Convert to the 24-hour clock.

18. 7:15 A.M. = _____   19. 3:30 P.M. = _____   20. 10:00 P.M. = _____

In the metric system, name the base units of:

Name	Abbreviation
(21) length	
(22) weight (mass)	
(23) substance	

Give the numerical value for each prefix.

24. deci _____

25. centi _____

26. milli _____

27. nano _____

28. micro _____

29. kilo _____

Do the following conversions of SI units:

30. 1 g = _____ mg

31. 1 L = _____ mL

32. 10 mg = _____ g

33. 1 kg = _____ g

34. 1 mg = _____ g

35. 250 mL = _____ L

36. 40 g = _____ kg

37. 200 mg = _____ g

38. 0.3 g = _____ mg

39. 1 m = _____ cm

40. 250 cm = _____ m

Your Score: /40 = %

Did you achieve 100%?

YES — Proceed to Module 4.

NO — Analyze your areas of weakness and review this module; then rewrite the post-test. If your score is still less than 100%, please seek remedial assistance.

Medication Orders and Dosage Forms

▶ MODULE TOPICS

- Reading of medication orders
- Commonly used abbreviations
- Packaging of medications
- Medication preparations
- Reading of medication labels

▶ INTRODUCTION

This module offers an opportunity to review common abbreviations in preparation for reading medication orders and medication labels. It is important to note that there are no standards for abbreviations; thus, these can vary between workplaces. Only those that are in common use and are not likely to be misinterpreted are used in this module. You are also provided with several examples of medication labels so that you can learn to locate necessary information and practise reading labels carefully. Again, no standards exist for the format, and you must become acquainted with various formats.

▶ READING OF MEDICATION ORDERS

All medication orders should include the patient's name, drug, dose, route, frequency or time of administration, date, and physician's signature.

CRITICAL POINT

The major cause of medication errors is misreading or misinterpretation of drug orders. Both calculating dosages and interpreting orders require 100% accuracy.

▶ COMMONLY USED ABBREVIATIONS

The first step in achieving accuracy of medication delivery is to correctly interpret the medication order. Handwriting jokes aside, even a legible order is usually written in shorthand. It's important to learn this "new language." Abbreviations vary considerably among institutions and among prescribers. Some are easily misinterpreted and can lead to error. For example, *qd* and *od* have been used to mean *daily* or *once a day*. However, *od* also means *right eye*. The abbreviation *qd* can also be confused with *qid*, which would result in a very serious error. For example, the drug digoxin (Lanoxin) would be given four times a day instead of only once. The letter *u*, meaning units, can be easily misread as an *o*. Serious drug errors have occurred because 6 u of insulin was read as 60. The abbreviations listed in Figure 4.1 have become widely accepted but are not standardized. Some have been used in the calculation problems in this workbook. You are urged to verify acceptable abbreviations used in your practice setting. For example, some settings use *DC* or *D/C* to mean *discontinue*, whereas other settings use these abbreviations to mean *discharge*.

ac	before meals
ad lib	as desired; freely
amp	ampule, ampoule
bid	twice daily
$\bar{c}$	with
cap	capsule
dil	dilute
/d	per day
elix	elixir
ext	extract
gtt	drop
h, hr	hour
hs	at bedtime
IM or im	intramuscular
inh	inhaler
I/O or I & O	intake & output (fluids)
IV or iv	intravenous
MAR	medication administration record
mcg	microgram
mEq	milliequivalent
mg	milligram
min	minute
N/G	nasogastric
OTC	over-the-counter
pc	after meals
PO or po	by mouth
PR	per rectum
prn	as necessary
qh	every hour
q4h	every 4 hours
qid	4 times a day
qs	as much as required
SC or sc	subcutaneous
SL or sl	sublingual
sol	solution
SR	slow or sustained release

(Continued)

FIGURE 4.1 Commonly Used Abbreviations

stat	immediately
supp	suppository
susp	suspension
tab	tablet
tid	3 times a day
IU or iu	international unit
ung	ointment
IVPB or ivpb	intravenous piggyback

FIGURE 4.1 *(Continued)*

NOTE: Sometimes these abbreviations are written with periods, for example, b.i.d., p.o. Well-known authors in the field of medication errors M.R. Cohen and N.M. Davis strongly advise against the use of certain abbreviations. For example *u*, for unit, has been mistaken for a *zero*, causing serious errors.

▶ EXERCISE 4.1

Complete the following exercise without referring to the above text. Correct your answers by using the answer guide starting on page 192.

PART I

Interpret the following medication orders. Write out each of the underlined abbreviations in full. (Value: 1 mark each)

1. meperidine (Demerol) 50–75 mg <u>IM q3–4h prn</u>
2. aluminum hydroxide 30 mL <u>po pc tid</u>
3. codeine sulfate 60 mg <u>PO stat and q4h</u>
4. penicillin G 500 000 units <u>IV qid</u>
5. phenobarbital <u>elix 100 mg hs</u>
6. insulin 6 units <u>sc stat</u>

Write in full the meaning for each of the following abbreviations. (Value: 1 mark each)

7. ad lib _____
8. gtt _____
9. SL _____
10. supp _____
11. pc _____
12. tab _____
13. bid _____
14. hs _____
15. ung _____
16. sc _____
17. ext _____

18. ac   _____
19. IM   _____
20. qs   _____
21. c̄   _____
22. stat   _____
23. sol   _____

Your Score: /23   =   %

PART II
Complete the crossword with the abbreviations. (Value: 17 marks)

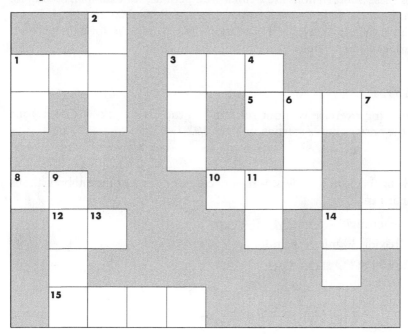

Across
1. as necessary
3. every 4 hours
5. immediately
8. after meals
10. twice daily
12. before meals
14. as much as required
15. suspension

Down
1. by mouth
2. ointment
3. 4 times a day
4. at bedtime
6. 3 times a day
7. tablets
9. capsules
11. intramuscular
14. every hour

Your Score: /17   =   %

▶ PACKAGING OF MEDICATIONS

Medications are prepared and packaged in a variety of forms. Oral doses are provided in compressed tablets, capsules, and liquids. Some tablets are scored and can be easily broken in half. Injectables are packaged in both single-dose and multiple-dose containers. Figures 4.2 and 4.3 illustrate various packaging of drugs.

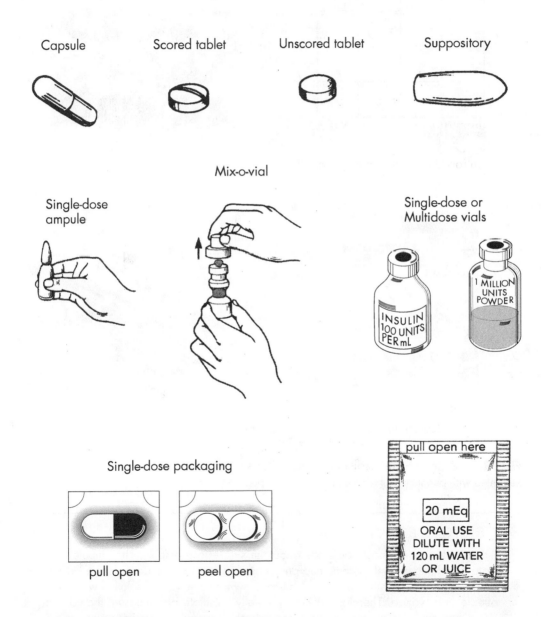

FIGURE 4.2 Packaging and dosage forms

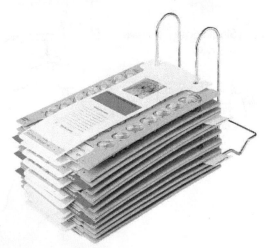

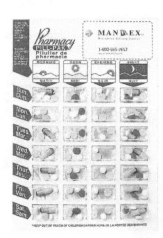

Controlled drug system (acute care)

Pill-Pak (community care)

Controlled dosage system (long-term care)

FIGURE 4.3 Unit-of-use medication packaging systems.
Reprinted with permission of Manrex Limited, Winnipeg, Manitoba.

CRITICAL POINT

An important point should be made about the single-dose ampule. The ampule may state that 1 mg per mL is contained and premixed for a single dose. However, the ampule contains slightly more than 1 mL to allow for some loss of solution within the needle and syringe. Therefore, always carefully calculate and measure the correct dose, and do not draw up the entire contents of an ampule. A similar point can be made regarding vials and bags of intravenous fluids. *All packages of liquid medication contain extra fluid.*

Injectables are prepared as liquids ready for injection or as powders requiring reconstitution with a diluent. The procedure for reconstitution and calculation of these products is described in Module 6.

▶ MEDICATION PREPARATIONS

As mentioned previously, medications may be prepared in tablets or capsules for oral administration, in liquid form for oral administration, and in solution for administration by parenteral routes (i.e., subcutaneous, intramuscular, and intravenous). In each of these forms, a certain weight of drug (e.g., milligrams) is contained in the product. Let's look at the labels in Figure 4.4 on page 54 to explain different forms of oral preparations. For example, in Figure 4.4A, the label states that 325 mg of acetaminophen is contained in one caplet. Therefore, the concentration of this drug product is 325 mg/cap. If a stronger preparation is desired, the caplet can be prepared in a greater concentration. Now see Figure 4.4B; the strength or concentration of this product is 500 mg/cap. Contrast these products with the one in Figure 4.4C. The strength of these chewable tablets is 160 mg/tab. If you were to arrange these drug forms from lowest to highest concentration (or strength), the order would be 160 mg/tab, 325 mg/cap, and 500 mg/cap. If the drug is required in a liquid preparation, a specific weight of drug is dissolved in a certain volume of liquid. See Figure 4.4D for an example; 80 mg of acetaminophen is dissolved in 1 mL of solution. The concentration is expressed as 80 mg/mL. As you will learn in the next section, reading medication labels carefully is very important. Now look at Figure 4.4E. What is the concentration of this drug product? It is 80 mg dissolved in 5 mL; therefore, the concentration is 16 mg/mL ($80 \div 5 = 16$). It is useful to think of all drug products as weight per volume, such as 325 mg/cap or 80 mg/mL.

Although many medications are weighed in milligrams, this is not true for all; for example, medications such as heparin, insulin, and penicillin are measured in units. The term *unit* refers to a drug measure based on a specific effect; for example, a unit of insulin is a standardized amount that lowers blood sugar. A few medications are measured in millimoles or milliequivalents. A mole is the gram molecular weight of a substance. A millimole is $\frac{1}{1000}$ of the mole. The term *milliequivalent* (mEq) refers to a measurement of combining power rather than weight. The equivalent weight is the gram weight of a substance that will combine with or replace 1 g of hydrogen. Sometimes the SI concentration (millimoles per litre) is the same as the conventional measure; for example, 95 mmol of chloride is equal to 95 mEq of chloride, and 4 mmol of potassium is equal to 4 mEq of potassium. In contrast, 2.4 mmol of magnesium is equal to 0.5 mEq of magnesium.

Here is a summary of important points regarding medication preparations:

- The strength or concentration of a drug is expressed as the weight of the drug in the dosage form, for example, *mg/tab* or *mg/mL*.
- The most common measure of weight is the milligram, but other measures such as units and milliequivalents are used for some specific drugs.
- Drugs may be prepared in solution.
  - A solution is a homogeneous mixture that contains one or more dissolved substances in a liquid. For example, when you add sugar to your tea, you are creating a solution.

A

COMPRIMÉS U.S.P.   TABLETS U.S.P.

ACÉTAMINOPHÈNE
ACETAMINOPHEN

325 MG

RÉGULIER / REGULAR

POUR SOULAGER LA DOULEUR
ET LA FIÈVRE
FOR RELIEF OF PAIN AND FEVER

120 CAPLETS   120 CAPLETS

DIN: 00789801

Il est peu probable que l'acétaminophène provoque des dérangements d'estomac ou de l'irritation gastrique. Il agit rapidement pour soulager temporairement les maux de tête, les douleurs musculaires, la douleur associée aux crampes menstruelles et la fièvre.

POSOLOGIE ORALE POUR ADULTES:
Prendre 1 ou 2 caplets et répéter à toutes les 4 heures au besoin. La dose quotidienne maximale est de 12 caplets ou tel que recommandé par le médecin. Il est dangereux de dépasser la dose maximale quotidienne recommandée sans consulter un médecin. Consulter un médecin si la situation exige l'usage continu pendant plus de 5 jours.
LIRE LE FEUILLET D'INFORMATION.

■ **MISE EN GARDE:** Ce contenant renferme suffisamment de médicaments pour être gravement nocif à un enfant.
CONSERVER CE MÉDICAMENT HORS DE LA PORTÉE DES ENFANTS.
BOUCHON SCELLÉ POUR VOTRE PROTECTION.

Acetaminophen is unlikely to cause stomach upset or gastric irritation and acts quickly to provide temporary relief from headaches, muscular aches, pain caused by menstrual cramps and fever.

ADULT ORAL DOSE:
Take 1 or 2 caplets, repeat every 4 hours if necessary. The maximum daily dose is 12 caplets or as recommended by a physician. It is hazardous to exceed the maximum recommended dose unless advised by a physician. Consult physician if the underlying condition requires continued use for more than 5 days.
READ DIRECTION CIRCULAR.

■ **CAUTION:** This package contains enough drug to seriously harm a child.
KEEP OUT OF REACH OF CHILDREN.
CAP SEALED FOR YOUR PROTECTION.

▲ LABORATOIRES TRIANON INC.
Trianon   BLAINVILLE (QUÉBEC) J7C 3V4

B

COMPRIMÉS U.S.P.   TABLETS U.S.P.

ACÉTAMINOPHÈNE
ACETAMINOPHEN

500 MG

EXTRA-FORT / EXTRA-STRENGTH

POUR SOULAGER LA DOULEUR
ET LA FIÈVRE
FOR RELIEF OF PAIN AND FEVER

120 CAPLETS   120 CAPLETS

DIN: 00789798

Il est peu probable que l'acétaminophène provoque des dérangements d'estomac ou de l'irritation gastrique. Il agit rapidement pour soulager temporairement les maux de tête, les douleurs musculaires, la douleur associée aux crampes menstruelles et la fièvre.

POSOLOGIE ORALE POUR ADULTES:
Prendre 1 ou 2 caplets et répéter à toutes les 4 heures au besoin. La dose quotidienne maximale est de 8 caplets ou tel que recommandé par le médecin. Il est dangereux de dépasser la dose maximale quotidienne recommandée sans consulter un médecin. Consulter un médecin si la situation exige l'usage continu pendant plus de 5 jours. Ce produit n'est pas un produit à doses normales et ne doit être utilisé que sur l'avis du médecin.

LIRE LE FEUILLET D'INFORMATION.

■ **MISE EN GARDE:** Ce contenant renferme suffisamment de médicaments pour être gravement nocif à un enfant.
CONSERVER CE MÉDICAMENT HORS DE LA PORTÉE DES ENFANTS.
BOUCHON SCELLÉ POUR VOTRE PROTECTION.

Acetaminophen is unlikely to cause stomach upset or gastric irritation and acts quickly to provide temporary relief from headaches, muscular aches, pain caused by menstrual cramps and fever.

ADULT ORAL DOSE:
Take 1 or 2 caplets, repeat every 4 hours if necessary. The maximum daily dose is 8 caplets as recommended by a physician. It is hazardous to exceed the maximum recommended dose unless advised by a physician. Consult physician if the underlying condition requires continued use for more than 5 days. This is not a normally dosaged product and should only be used on the advice of a physician.

READ DIRECTION CIRCULAR.

■ **CAUTION:** This package contains enough drug to seriously harm a child.
KEEP OUT OF REACH OF CHILDREN.
CAP SEALED FOR YOUR PROTECTION.

▲ LABORATOIRES TRIANON INC.
Trianon   BLAINVILLE (QUÉBEC) J7C 3V4

C

COMPRIMÉS CROQUABLES
D'ACÉTAMINOPHÈNE
U.S.P. POUR ENFANTS
ACETAMINOPHEN
CHEWABLE TABLETS U.S.P.
FOR CHILDREN
20 comprimés/tablets
160 mg

DIN 02017431

Chaque comprimé croquable contient 160mg d'acétaminophène.
Pour le soulagement rapide de la fièvre et de la douleur légère dues aux immunisations, la dentition ou la grippe chez les enfants.
Posologie: Administrer une seule dose selon l'âge (voir ci-dessous) toutes les 4 heures jusqu'à un maximum quotidien de 5 doses ou selon les indications du médecin.

ÂGE	DOSE UNIQUE MAXIMALE	
Enfants de moins de 2 (deux) ans: selon les indications du médecin		
2 à 3 ans	1 comprimé	(160mg)
4 à 5 ans	1 ½ comprimé	(240mg)
6 à 8 ans	2 comprimés	(320mg)
9 à 10 ans	2 ½ comprimés	(400mg)
11 à 12 ans	3 comprimés	(480mg)

Il est dangereux de dépasser la dose recommandée (voir feuillet à l'intérieur) sans l'avis d'un médecin. Si l'état pathologique sous-jacent de l'enfant persiste durant plus de 5 jours, consulter un médecin.
Les ingrédients inactifs figurent sur la boîte.
Le bouchon est scellé pour votre sécurité. Emballage protège-enfant.
■ **CONSERVER CE MÉDICAMENT HORS DE LA PORTÉE DES ENFANTS**

Each chewable tablet contains 160mg of acetaminophen.
For fast relief from fever and minor pain due to immunizations, teething or flu for children.
Dosage: Administer single dose according to age as listed below, every 4 hours, to a maximum of 5 times daily or as directed by a physician.

AGE	MAXIMUM SINGLE DOSE	
Under 2 (two) years: as directed by a physician.		
2 to 3 years	1 tablet	(160mg)
4 to 5 years	1 ½ tablet	(240mg)
6 to 8 years	2 tablets	(320mg)
9 to 10 years	2 ½ tablets	(400mg)
11 to 12 years	3 tablets	(480mg)

It is hazardous to exceed the recommended dosage, unless advised by a physician (see instruction sheet inside). If underlying condition persists for more than 5 days, consult a physician.
For inactive ingredients, see outer carton.
The cap is **sealed for your protection.** Child resistant package.
■ **KEEP THIS MEDICATION OUT OF REACH OF CHILDREN**

LABORATOIRE RHA INC.   BLAINVILLE (QUÉBEC) CANADA J7C 3V4

D

SOLUTION ORALE
D'ACÉTAMINOPHÈNE
U.S.P.
ACETAMINOPHEN
ORAL SOLUTION

GOUTTES / DROPS

80 MG / ML • 15 ML

DIN 01905864

Chaque ml contient 80 mg d'acétaminophène.
Pour le soulagement rapide de la fièvre et de la douleur chez les enfants.
POSOLOGIE: Administrer une seule dose selon l'âge (voir liste ci-dessous) toutes les 4 heures, jusqu'à un maximum de 5 doses par jour ou selon les recommandations du médecin. L'emballage contient un compte-gouttes gradué de 0.5 ml.

ÂGE	DOSE UNIQUE MAXIMALE
0 à 3 mois	0.5 ml. (40 mg)
4 à 11 mois	1.0 ml. (80 mg)
12 à 23 mois	1.5 ml. (120 mg)
2 et 3 ans	2.0 ml. (160 mg)
4 et 5 ans	3.0 ml. (240 mg)

Solution Concentrée
Il est dangereux de dépasser la dose recommandée (voir le feuillet à l'intérieur) sans l'avis d'un médecin. Si l'état pathologique sous-jacent de l'enfant persiste durant plus de 5 jours, consulter un médecin.
LIRE LE FEUILLET D'INFORMATION.

Bouchon scellé pour votre sécurité.
Contenant à l'épreuve des enfants.

■ **CONSERVER CE MÉDICAMENT HORS DE LA PORTÉE DES ENFANTS.**

Each ml contains 80 mg of acetaminophen.
For fast effective relief of pain and fever in children.
DOSAGE: Administer a single dose according to age (see list below) every 4 hours, up to 5 times a day or as directed by the physician. With 0.5 ml graduated dropper.

AGE	MAXIMUM SINGLE DOSE
0 to 3 months	0.5 mL (40 mg)
4 to 11 months	1.0 mL (80 mg)
12 to 23 months	1.5 mL (120 mg)
2 and 3 years	2.0 mL (160 mg)
4 and 5 years	3.0 mL (240 mg)

Concentrate Solution
It is hazardous to exceed the recommended dosage (see package insert) except on the advice of a physician. If the underlying condition persists for more than 5 days, consult a physician.
READ DIRECTION CIRCULAR.

Cap sealed for your protection.
Child resistant package.

■ **KEEP THIS MEDICATION OUT OF THE REACH OF CHILDREN.**

▲ LABORATOIRES TRIANON INC.
Trianon   BLAINVILLE (QUÉBEC) J7C 3V4

E

SOLUTION ORALE
D'ACÉTAMINOPHÈNE
U.S.P. POUR ENFANTS
CHILDREN'S
ACETAMINOPHEN
ORAL SOLUTION U.S.P.

SOULAGEMENT DE LA FIÈVRE ET DE LA
DOULEUR CHEZ LES ENFANTS
FAST RELIEF OF CHILDREN'S FEVER AND PAIN

80 MG / 5 ML • 100 ML

DIN 01905848

Une cuillère à thé (5 ml) contient 80 mg d'acétaminophène.
Pour le soulagement rapide de la fièvre et de la douleur légère occasionnées par l'immunisation, la dentition, le rhume chez les enfants et les nourrissons.
POSOLOGIE: Administrer une seule dose selon l'âge (voir liste ci-dessous) toutes les 4 heures, jusqu'à un maximum de 5 doses par jour ou selon les recommandations du médecin.

ÂGE	DOSE UNIQUE MAXIMALE
Enfants de 2 ans:	selon les recommandations du médecin.
2 ans à 4 ans	2 c. à thé (10 ml)
4 ans à 6 ans	3 c. à thé (15 ml)
6 ans à 9 ans	4 c. à thé (20 ml)
9 ans à 11 ans	5 c. à thé (25 ml)
11 ans à 12 ans	6 c. à thé (30 ml)

Il est dangereux de dépasser la dose recommandée (voir le feuillet à l'intérieur) sans l'avis d'un médecin. Si l'état pathologique sous-jacent de l'enfant persiste durant plus de 5 jours, consulter un médecin.
LIRE LE FEUILLET D'INFORMATION.

Bouchon scellé pour votre sécurité.
Contenant à l'épreuve des enfants.

■ **CONSERVER CE MÉDICAMENT HORS DE LA PORTÉE DES ENFANTS.**

One teaspoonful (5 ml) contains 80 mg of acetaminophen.
For fast relief of fever and minor pain due to immunizations, teething and flu in children and infants.
DOSAGE: Administer a single dose according to age (see list below) every 4 hours, up to 5 times a day or as directed by the physician.

AGE	MAXIMUM SINGLE DOSE
Children 2 years:	as directed by a physician.
2 to 4 years	2 teaspoonful (10 ml)
4 to 6 years	3 teaspoonful (15 ml)
6 to 9 years	4 teaspoonful (20 ml)
9 to 11 years	5 teaspoonful (25 ml)
11 to 12 years	6 teaspoonful (30 ml)

It is hazardous to exceed the recommended dosage (see package insert) except on the advice of a physician. If the underlying condition persists for more than 5 days, consult a physician.
READ DIRECTION CIRCULAR.

Cap sealed for your protection. Child resistant package.

■ **KEEP THIS MEDICATION OUT OF THE REACH OF CHILDREN.**

▲ LABORATOIRES TRIANON INC.
Trianon   BLAINVILLE (QUÉBEC) J7C 3V4

FIGURE 4.4
Trianon Laboratories Inc., Blainville, Quebec.

- A solvent is the liquid in which another substance is dissolved. In the above example, the tea is the solvent.
- A solute is the substance that is dissolved in the solvent. In our example, sugar is the solute.
- There are two types of solutions: weight-per-volume solutions and volume-per-volume solutions.
  - In a weight-per-volume solution, the solute is weighed and the solvent is expressed in volume. This is the most common type of medication solution. For example, see the label in Figure 4.5 on page 56. The label states that 25 g of dextrose is dissolved in 50 mL (of sterile water). Therefore, the concentration of the solution is 500 mg/mL (25 g = 25 000 mg; 25 000 mg in 50 mL = 500 mg per mL).
  - In a volume-per-volume solution, both the solute and the solvent are measured in the same units of volume. For example, 1 mL of drug is added to 25 mL of intravenous solution.
- The medication label indicates the strength (or concentration) of the drug. The strength may be stated as a percentage. For example, in Figure 4.5, the label states "Dextrose 50%." A 1% solution has 1 g of drug in 100 mL of solvent; therefore, a 50% solution has 50 g in 100 mL. Note that the product in Figure 4.5 is only 50 mL; therefore, 25 g are dissolved in 50 mL. (You can use proportion to prove this statement.)
- The strength of a drug solution may also be stated as a ratio. If the label states 1:1000, this means that 1 g of drug is dissolved in 1000 mL (or that the strength is 1 mg per mL). For example, view the label in Figure 4.6 on page 57. Note that it is described as 1:10 000; this means that 1 g of drug is dissolved in 10 000 mL (or that the strength is 0.1 mg per mL).

▶ EXERCISE 4.2

Complete the following exercise without referring to the above text. Correct your answers by using the answer guide starting on page 192. (Value: 1 mark each)

Complete each of the following sentences with the most appropriate term.

1. A homogeneous mixture that contains one or more dissolved substances in a liquid is called a _____ .

2. The substance that is dissolved in a solution is called a _____ .

3. In a solution, the liquid in which a substance is dissolved is called a _____ .

For questions 4 and 5, choose the correct answer.

4. Which solution has the greater concentration?
   a. 1000 units per 1 mL
   b. 10 000 units per 1 mL

5. The labels on two vials of the same medication indicate that the concentrations are:
   Drug A: 10 mg/mL
   Drug B: 100 mg in 10 mL
   Is the concentration of Drug A:
   a. the same as that of Drug B?

b. less than that of Drug B?

c. greater than that of Drug B?

Answer questions 6 to 9 by indicating the unit of measurement for the solute and the solvent for each type of solution. Choose your response from this list of units: gram, milligram, or millilitre.

6. In a weight-per-volume solution, the unit of measurement of the solute is a
_____.

7. In a weight-per-volume solution, the unit of measurement of the solvent is a
_____.

8. In a volume-per-volume solution, the unit of measurement of the solute is a
_____.

9. In a volume-per-volume solution, the unit of measurement of the solvent is a
_____.

In questions 10 and 11, indicate whether the solutions are weight-per-volume or volume-per-volume.

10. A solution that has 5 g of solute, pure drug, dissolved in 100 mL of solvent is termed a _____ solution.

11. You have mixed 5 mL of lemon juice with 250 mL of water. You have prepared a _____ solution.

Study the label in Figure 4.5 and answer questions 12 to 14.

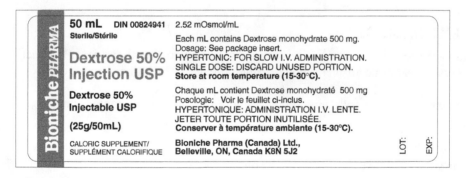

FIGURE 4.5
Bioniche Pharma Group, London, Ontario.

12. The drug product is a solution. State the concentration of the solution in milligrams per millilitre.

13. Explain what is meant by a 50% solution.

14. How many grams of drug (dextrose) would be contained in 10 mL of this solution?

Study the label in Figure 4.6 and answer questions 15 and 16.

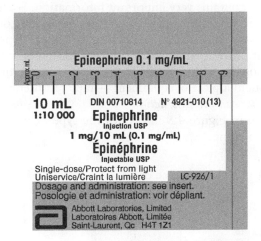

FIGURE 4.6
Reprinted with permission of Abbott Laboratories Limited, Montreal, Quebec.

15. Explain what is meant by a solution that is labelled 1:10 000.
16. State the concentration of the drug in milligrams per millilitre.

Study the label in Figure 4.7 and answer questions 17 to 20.

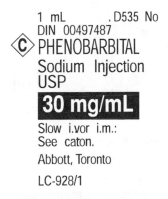

FIGURE 4.7
Reprinted with permission of Abbott Laboratories Limited, Montreal, Quebec.

17. In this drug solution, name the solute.
18. State the concentration of this drug solution.
19. How much drug would be contained in 0.5 mL?
20. State the strength of this solution, as a percentage. Recall that a 1% solution has 1 g of drug dissolved in 100 mL of solvent.

| Your Score: | /20 | = | % |

▶ READING OF MEDICATION LABELS

The medication label contains very important information. Some labels are clearly presented, provided your vision is satisfactory! Other labels are confusing. Labels are not standardized as to what information is included or how it is presented. It's important to develop the habit of thoroughly studying the information and instructions on drug labels. Accompanying literature also provides useful information. Check your habits: the last time you bought a piece of equipment — tape recorder, video machine, or pocket calculator — *did you read the instructions?*

The label shown in Figure 4.8 illustrates the type of information that should be included in drug packaging.

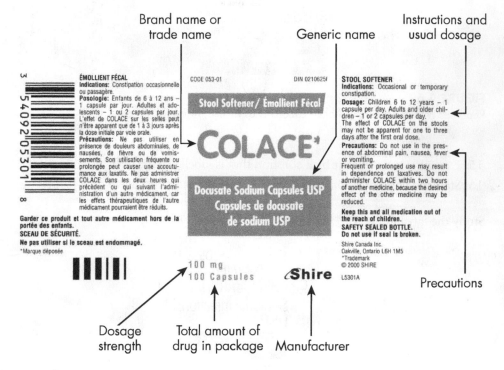

FIGURE 4.8 Reading a medication label.
WellSpring Pharmaceutical Canada Corp., Oakville, Ontario.

The brand or trade name is given by a manufacturer. The generic name is a brief form of the chemical name of the drug. The same generic drug may be sold under different brand or trade names. A certain brand name may not be available in different countries. For example, the generic chlorpromazine is available as Largactil in Canada and Thorazine in the United States. It is important to learn both the generic and the trade names; sometimes the medication order states one name and the label on the product gives the other.

NOTE: This book does not teach you the drug names, but it uses actual names (both generic and trade) in the labels and orders that are provided for you to practise reading. See Appendix C for examples of brand names used in Canada, Australia, and the United States.

CRITICAL POINT

Medication labels are not standardized. You must read labels very carefully, as illustrated by the following example. The same drug is supplied in three dosage forms. The first is a 2-mL ampule labelled 20 mcg/mL; the second is a 2-mL ampule labelled 1 mg/mL. Note the difference in the strength of the product in the two ampules. Using medication from the wrong ampule could result in serious consequences. The third dosage form is a 10-mL vial labelled 4 mg. Since 4 mg is contained in the vial, and the total volume is 10 mL, the concentration is 4 mg/10 mL or 0.4 mg/mL.

▶ **EXERCISE 4.3**

Complete the following exercise without referring to the above text. Correct your answers by using the answer guide starting on page 192. (Value: 1 mark each)

Study the label in Figure 4.9 and answer questions 1 to 6.

ÉMOLLIENT FÉCAL
Indications: Constipation occasionelle ou passagère.
Posologie: Administrer dans un demi-verre (120mL) de lait ou de jus de fruit ou dans une préparation pour nourrissons. Nourrissons et enfants de moins de 3 ans – selon les directives du médecin. **Enfants de 3 à 6 ans** – 2 mL une à trois fois par jour, jusqu'à ce que l'évacuation des selles revienne à la normale. L'effet de COLACE sur les selles peut n'être apparent que de 1 à 3 jours après la dose initiale par voie orale.
Garder ce produit et tout autre médicament hors de la portée des enfants.
SCEAU DE SÉCURITÉ
Précautions: VOIR LA BOÎTE
*Marque déposée
L4163B

CODE 416-30   DIN 02090163

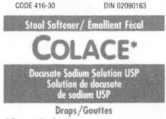
Stool Softener/ Émollient Fécal
COLACE*
Docusate Sodium Solution USP
Solution de docusate
de sodium USP
Drops/Gouttes
1 0 m g / m L
3 0 m L

STOOL SOFTENER
Indications: Occasional or temporary constipation.
Dosage: Add drops to one-half glassful (120mL) of milk, fruit juice or infant's formula. Infants and children under 3 – as prescribed by physician. **Children 3 to 6 years** – 2 mL one to three times daily until bowel movements are normal.
The effect of COLACE on the stools may not be apparent for one to three days after the first oral dose.
Keep this and all medication out of the reach of children.
SAFETY FEATURE: BANDED CAP
Precautions: SEE CARTON
Shire Canada Inc.
Oakville, Ontario L6H 1M5
*Trademark
©2000 Shire

FIGURE 4.9
WellSpring Pharmaceutical Canada Corp., Oakville, Ontario.

1. State the form of the drug.
2. What is the dosage strength?
3. State the trade drug name.
4. State the generic drug name.
5. State the usual dose for children 3 to 6 years.
6. What is the total volume (in millilitres)?

Study the label in Figure 4.10 and answer questions 7 to 10.

5 mL

Heparin Leo*

Heparin Sodium Injection B.P.
Héparine sodique injectable B.P.

10,000 i.u./mL

I.V./S.C.

DIN: 00579718

L E O
*Regd User
Leo Pharma Inc.,
Thornhill, Ontario

006176-02

FIGURE 4.10
Leo Pharma Inc., Thornhill, Ontario.

7. What is the total amount of heparin sodium contained in this multidose vial?
8. What is the concentration of the heparin sodium solution?
9. Name the solute in this solution.
10. What is the total volume contained in the vial?

Your Score: /10 = %

▶ **EXERCISE 4.4**

Complete the following exercise without referring to the above text. Correct your answers by using the answer guide starting on page 192. (Value: 1 mark each)

Study the labels in Figure 4.11 and answer questions 1 to 10.

A. **Usual adult dosage:** Titration begins with 5 mg 3 times a day for 3 days, followed by increases to 10, 15, and 20 mg 3 times a day at 3-day intervals. Maximum dose should not exceed 80 mg daily (20 mg 4 times a day). Not recommended in children. If benefits are not evident after a trial period, the medication should be *withdrawn slowly*. Product monograph supplied on request. Protect from heat and humidity.

Novartis Pharmaceuticals Canada Inc.
Novartis Pharma Canada inc.
Dorval (Québec) H9S 1A9

3349-11-00A

Lioresal®10mg
baclofen tablets USP
comprimés de baclofène USP

DIN 00455881   1635

Ⓤ NOVARTIS

Muscle relaxant, antispastic
Relaxant musculaire, antispastique

100 tablets
100 comprimés

Posologie habituelle pour adulte : Instituer le traitement avec 5 mg 3 fois par jour pour 3 jours; augmenter la dose à 10, 15, et 20 mg 3 fois par jour à 3 jours d'intervalle. La dose maximale ne devrait pas dépasser 80 mg par jour (20 mg 4 fois par jour). L'emploi chez l'enfant n'est pas conseillé. Si après une période d'essai la réponse n'est pas satisfaisante, *le sevrage devrait se faire lentement.* Monographie fournie sur demande. Protéger de la chaleur et de l'humidité.

0 63601 01635 1

B. **Usual Adult Dosage:** Titration begins with 5 mg 3 times a day for 3 days, followed by increases to 10, 15 and 20 mg 3 times a day at 3-day intervals. Maximum dose should not exceed 80 mg daily (20 mg 4 times a day). Not recommended in children. If benefits are not evident after a trial period, the medication should be *withdrawn slowly*. Product monograph supplied on request. Protect from heat and humidity.

Novartis Pharmaceuticals Canada Inc.
Novartis Pharma Canada inc.
Dorval (Québec) H9S 1A9

3368-11-00A

Lioresal®D.S. 20mg
baclofen tablets USP
comprimés de baclofène USP

DIN 00636576   1640

Ⓤ NOVARTIS

Muscle relaxant, antispastic
Relaxant musculaire, antispastique

100 tablets
100 comprimés

Posologie habituelle pour adulte : Instituer le traitement avec 5 mg 3 fois par jour pour 3 jours; augmenter la dose à 10, 15 et 20 mg 3 fois par jour à 3 jours d'intervalle. La dose maximale ne devrait pas dépasser 80 mg par jour (20 mg 4 fois par jour). L'emploi chez l'enfant n'est pas conseillé. Si après une période d'essai la réponse n'est pas satisfaisante, *le sevrage devrait se faire lentement.* Monographie fournie sur demande. Protéger de la chaleur et de l'humidité.

0 63601 01640 5

FIGURE 4.11
Novartis Pharmaceuticals Canada Inc., Dorval, Quebec.

1. State the trade or brand name of the drug.
2. State the generic name of the drug.
3. Refer to Figure 4.11A. State the concentration of the drug.
4. Refer to Figure 4.11B. State the concentration of the drug.
5. Refer to either label and state the usual adult dose.
6. How many tablets are contained in each of these bottles?
7. According to the label, what is this drug used for (what is the class of drug)?
8. What is the name of the manufacturer?
9. Refer to Figure 4.11A. If an individual takes 3 tablets per day, how long would this supply last?
10. Which of the 2 products in Figure 4.11 has the greatest concentration?

Your Score:	/10	=	%

▶ EXERCISE 4.5

Complete the following exercise without referring to the above text. Correct your answers by using the answer guide starting on page 192. (Value: 1 mark each)

Study the labels in Figure 4.12 and answer questions 1 to 15.

1. State the generic name of the drug.
2. What is the recommended use of the drug?
3. Refer to Figure 4.12A. State the dosage concentration of the drug in milligrams per millilitre.
4. Refer to Figure 4.12B. State the dosage concentration of the drug in milligrams per millilitre.
5. Refer to Figure 4.12C. State the dosage concentration of the drug in milligrams per millilitre.
6. Refer to Figure 4.12A. State the total volume in the bottle.
7. Refer to Figure 4.12B. State the total volume in the bottle.
8. Refer to Figure 4.12C. State the total volume in the bottle.
9. Refer to Figure 4.12A. Find the recommended maximum single dose for an 18-month-old infant.
10. Refer to Figures 4.12A and B. What device should be used to administer the medication?
11. Which product has the weakest concentration?
12. What is the name of the manufacturer?
13. Refer to Figure 4.12C. Find the recommended dose for a 7-year-old child; express it in milligrams.
14. Refer to Figure 4.12C. If a 12-year-old took the recommended dose, how many doses would this bottle provide?

15. Refer to Figure 4.12C. A mother gave her 6-year-old child 2 tsp. of this solution. Is this within the recommended dose?

Your Score: /15 = %

A

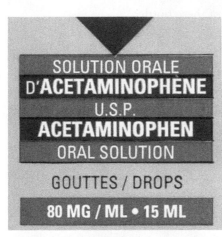

SOLUTION ORALE
D'ACÉTAMINOPHÈNE
U.S.P.
ACETAMINOPHEN
ORAL SOLUTION

GOUTTES / DROPS

80 MG / ML • 15 ML

DIN 01905864

Chaque ml contient 80 mg d'acétaminophène.
Pour le soulagement rapide de la fièvre et de la douleur chez les enfants.
POSOLOGIE: Administrer une seule dose selon l'âge (voir liste ci-dessous) toutes les 4 heures, jusqu'à un maximum de 5 doses par jour ou selon les recommandations du médecin. L'emballage contient un compte-gouttes gradué de 0.5 ml.

ÂGE	DOSE UNIQUE MAXIMALE
0 à 3 mois	0.5 mL (40 mg)
4 à 11 mois	1.0 mL (80 mg)
12 à 23 mois	1.5 mL (120 mg)
2 et 3 ans	2.0 mL (160 mg)
4 et 5 ans	3.0 mL (240 mg)

Solution Concentrée
Il est dangereux de dépasser la dose recommandée (voir le feuillet à l'intérieur) sans l'avis d'un médecin. Si l'état pathologique sous-jacent de l'enfant persiste durant plus de 5 jours, consulter un médecin.
LIRE LE FEUILLET D'INFORMATION.
Bouchon scellé pour votre sécurité.
Contenant à l'épreuve des enfants.

CONSERVER CE MÉDICAMENT HORS DE LA PORTÉE DES ENFANTS.

Each ml contains 80 mg of acetaminophen.
For fast effective relief of pain and fever in children.
DOSAGE: Administer a single dose according to age (see list below) every 4 hours, up to 5 times a day or as directed by the physician. With 0.5 ml graduated dropper.

AGE	MAXIMUM SINGLE DOSE
0 to 3 months	0.5 mL (40 mg)
4 to 11 months	1.0 mL (80 mg)
12 to 23 months	1.5 mL (120 mg)
2 and 3 years	2.0 mL (160 mg)
4 and 5 years	3.0 mL (240 mg)

Concentrate Solution
It is hazardous to exceed the recommended dosage (see package insert) except on the advice of a physician. If the underlying condition persists for more than 5 days, consult a physician.
READ DIRECTION CIRCULAR.
Cap sealed for your protection.
Child resistant package.

KEEP THIS MEDICATION OUT OF THE REACH OF CHILDREN.

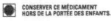
LABORATOIRES TRIANON INC. BLAINVILLE (QUÉBEC) J7C 3V4

B

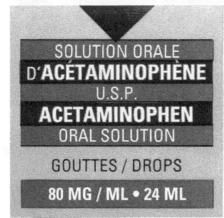

SOLUTION ORALE
D'ACÉTAMINOPHÈNE
U.S.P.
ACETAMINOPHEN
ORAL SOLUTION

GOUTTES / DROPS

80 MG / ML • 24 ML

DIN 01905864

Chaque ml contient 80 mg d'acétaminophène.
Pour le soulagement rapide de la fièvre et de la douleur chez les enfants.
POSOLOGIE: Administrer une seule dose selon l'âge (voir liste ci-dessous) toutes les 4 heures, jusqu'à un maximum de 5 doses par jour ou selon les recommandations du médecin. L'emballage contient un compte-gouttes gradué de 0.5 ml.

ÂGE	DOSE UNIQUE MAXIMALE
0 à 3 mois	0.5 mL (40 mg)
4 à 11 mois	1.0 mL (80 mg)
12 à 23 mois	1.5 mL (120 mg)
2 et 3 ans	2.0 mL (160 mg)
4 et 5 ans	3.0 mL (240 mg)

Solution Concentrée
Il est dangereux de dépasser la dose recommandée (voir le feuillet à l'intérieur) sans l'avis d'un médecin. Si l'état pathologique sous-jacent de l'enfant persiste durant plus de 5 jours, consulter un médecin.
LIRE LE FEUILLET D'INFORMATION.
Bouchon scellé pour votre sécurité.
Contenant à l'épreuve des enfants.

CONSERVER CE MÉDICAMENT HORS DE LA PORTÉE DES ENFANTS.

Each ml contains 80 mg of acetaminophen.
For fast effective relief of pain and fever in children.
DOSAGE: Administer a single dose according to age (see list below) every 4 hours, up to 5 times a day or as directed by the physician. With 0.5 ml graduated dropper.

AGE	MAXIMUM SINGLE DOSE
0 to 3 months	0.5 mL (40 mg)
4 to 11 months	1.0 mL (80 mg)
12 to 23 months	1.5 mL (120 mg)
2 and 3 years	2.0 mL (160 mg)
4 and 5 years	3.0 mL (240 mg)

Concentrate Solution
It is hazardous to exceed the recommended dosage (see package insert) except on the advice of a physician. If the underlying condition persists for more than 5 days, consult a physician.
READ DIRECTION CIRCULAR.
Cap sealed for your protection.
Child resistant package.

KEEP THIS MEDICATION OUT OF THE REACH OF CHILDREN.

LABORATOIRES TRIANON INC. BLAINVILLE (QUÉBEC) J7C 3V4

C

SOLUTION ORALE
D'ACÉTAMINOPHÈNE
U.S.P. POUR ENFANTS
CHILDREN'S
ACETAMINOPHEN
ORAL SOLUTION U.S.P.

SOULAGEMENT DE LA FIÈVRE ET DE LA DOULEUR CHEZ LES ENFANTS
FAST RELIEF OF CHILDREN'S FEVER AND PAIN

160 MG / 5 ML • 100 ML

DIN 01955536

Une cuillerée à thé (5 ml) contient 160 mg d'acétaminophène.
Pour le soulagement rapide de la fièvre et de la douleur légère occasionnées par l'immunisation, la dentition, la grippe chez les enfants.
POSOLOGIE: Administrer une seule dose selon l'âge (voir liste ci-dessous) toutes les 4 heures, jusqu'à un maximum de 5 doses par jour ou selon les recommandations du médecin.

ÂGE	DOSE UNIQUE MAXIMALE
Enfants de 2 ans:	selon les recommandations du médecin.
2 ans à 4 ans	1 c. à thé (5 ml)
4 ans à 6 ans	1½ c. à thé (7.5 ml)
6 ans à 9 ans	2 c. à thé (10 ml)
9 ans à 11 ans	2½ c. à thé (12.5 ml)
11 ans à 12 ans	3 c. à thé (15 ml)

Il est dangereux de dépasser la dose recommandée (voir le feuillet à l'intérieur) sans l'avis d'un médecin. Si l'état pathologique sous-jacent de l'enfant persiste durant plus de 5 jours, consulter un médecin.
LIRE LE FEUILLET D'INFORMATION.
Bouchon scellé pour votre sécurité.
Contenant à l'épreuve des enfants.

CONSERVER CE MÉDICAMENT HORS DE LA PORTÉE DES ENFANTS.

One teaspoonful (5 ml) contains 160 mg of acetaminophen.
For fast relief of fever and minor pain due to immunizations, teething and flu in children.
DOSAGE: Administer a single dose according to age (see list below) every 4 hours, up to 5 times a day or as directed by the physician.

AGE	MAXIMUM SINGLE DOSE
Children 2 years:	as directed by a physician.
2 to 4 years	1 teaspoonful (5 ml)
4 to 6 years	1½ teaspoonful (7.5 ml)
6 to 9 years	2 teaspoonful (10 ml)
9 to 11 years	2½ teaspoonful (12.5 ml)
11 to 12 years	3 teaspoonful (15 ml)

It is hazardous to exceed the recommended dosage (see package insert) except on the advice of a physician. If the underlying condition persists for more than 5 days, consult a physician.
READ DIRECTION CIRCULAR.
Cap sealed for your protection. Child resistant package.

KEEP THIS MEDICATION OUT OF THE REACH OF CHILDREN.

LABORATOIRES TRIANON INC. BLAINVILLE (QUÉBEC) J7C 3V4

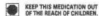

FIGURE 4.12
Trianon Laboratories Inc., Blainville, Quebec.

▶ EXERCISE 4.6

Complete the following exercise without referring to the above text. Correct your answers by using the answer guide starting on page 192. (Value: 1 mark each)

Interpret the medication orders in questions 1 to 5. Write out each of the underlined abbreviations in full.

1. chloral hydrate 750 <u>mg hs prn</u>
2. potassium chloride 20 <u>mEq bid IV</u>
3. dexamethasone 2 <u>mg PO tid</u>
4. RhoGAM 300 <u>mcg IM</u>
5. fentanyl citrate 0.8 <u>mcg/kg IV stat</u>
6. If you add milk to tea, what type of solution have you created?
7. If you add sugar to coffee, what type of solution have you created?
8. Complete the following sentence: A 5% solution has ___ g of medication in every ____ mL of solution.
9. A label reads, "10% solution." How many grams of medication are dissolved in 100 mL of solution?

Read the following statement and answer questions 10 to 12: A drug is prepared in two strengths. One label indicates a 1:1000 ratio, and the other label indicates 1:10 000.

10. Which product has the greatest concentration?
11. Express the drug concentration in milligrams per millilitre for each product.
12. In the product with the greatest concentration, how much drug would be contained in 0.6 mL?

Complete the chart; an example is provided. Round to the nearest hundredth.

Drug Product	Concentration (per mL)
haloperidol (Haldol) multidose vial = 5 mL vial contains 250 mg	250 mg/5 mL = 50 mg/mL
furosemide (Lasix) single-dose vial = 4 mL vial contains 40 mg	(13)
acetaminophen oral drops multidose bottle = 24 mL bottle contains 1920 mg	(14)
potassium chloride elixir 1 tbsp. = 40 mEq	(15)

Your Score:	/15	=	%

▶ OPTIONAL ACTIVITY

Reading labels requires practice and attention. Learning where to find the information comes with experience. This book cannot provide enough situations to practise, so you are encouraged to do any of the following activities to become familiar with drug product forms and labels.

1. Visit a drugstore. Browse and read labels. Look for generic and trade names, the forms of the drugs, dosage strengths, the number of tablets supplied, usual recommended doses, and other ingredients (e.g., preservatives, colouring).

2. Ask your clinical instructor or preceptor to show you various drug products in the clinical setting. Become familiar with the variety of labels, and, again, look on each label for the name (generic and trade), other ingredients, drug form and strength, storage instructions, recommended dose, and administration precautions.

▶ POST-TEST

Instructions

1. Write the post-test without referring to any resources.

2. Correct the post-test by using the answer guide starting on page 192.

PART I

Match the abbreviation in column 1 with the correct expression in column 2. (Value: 1 mark each)

Column 1

1. stat ____
2. pc ____
3. ung ____
4. elix ____
5. ac ____
6. tab ____
7. bid ____
8. cap ____
9. hs ____
10. sc ____

Column 2

A. twice daily
B. capsule
C. ointment
D. at bedtime
E. after meals
F. elixir
G. subcutaneous
H. tablet
I. before meals
J. immediately

PART II

Study the label in Figure 4.13 and answer questions 1 to 6. (Value: 1 mark each)

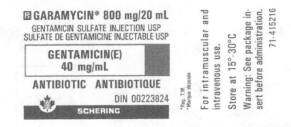

FIGURE 4.13
Schering Canada Inc., Pointe-Claire, Quebec.

1. What is the form of the drug?
2. What is the trade name of the drug?
3. What is the generic name of the drug?
4. What is the concentration of the drug?
5. What are the routes of administration?
6. What is the total volume?

PART III

Rewrite the following orders with the abbreviations expanded. (Value: 1 mark each)

1. prednisone 30 mg PO × 3 days
2. digoxin 250 mcg PO daily
3. demerol 75 mg IM q3–4h prn
4. nitroglycerin spray SL prn
5. nifedipine tab 20 mg PO bid
6. glycerin supp PR prn
7. salbutamol inh 100 mcg/dose, 2 puffs q4–6h
8. insulin 10 units SC stat
9. antibiotic by ivpb
10. cough elix qs

PART IV

Answer questions 1 to 4. (Value: 1 mark each)

1. Which solution has the greater concentration?
   a. 1000 units per mL
   b. 10 000 units per mL
2. Complete the following sentence: A 10% solution has 10 g of drug dissolved in _____ mL of solution.
3. The label states, "1:1000." What does this mean?
4. In the previous question, what is the strength of the solution expressed as milligrams per millilitre?

PART V

Study the label in Figure 4.14 and answer questions 1 to 5. (Value: 1 mark each)

10x 1mL

Heparin Leo*
Heparin Sodium Injection B.P.
Héparine sodique injectable B.P.

DIN: 00579718

10,000 i.u./mL

ANTICOAGULANT
Injection I.V./S.C.

*Regd User
Leo Pharma Inc.,
Thornhill, Ontario

Heparin Leo*   10,000 i.u./mL

FIGURE 4.14
Leo Pharma Inc., Thornhill, Ontario.

1. State the trade name of the drug.
2. State the generic name of the drug.
3. Identify the manufacturer.
4. State the concentration of the drug product.
5. What routes of administration can be used with this drug form?

Total Score

Part I: _____ /10 = _____ %

Part II: _____ /6 = _____ %

Part III: _____ /10 = _____ %

Part IV: _____ /4 = _____ %

Part V: _____ /5 = _____ %

Your Score: /35   =   %

Did you achieve 100%?

YES — Proceed to Module 5.

NO — Analyze your areas of weakness and review this module; then rewrite the post-test.
If your score is still less than 100%, please seek remedial assistance.

Calculation of Oral Medication Doses

▶ MODULE TOPICS

- Definitions
- Use of a calculator
  - Calculation of decimals
  - Calculation of fractions
- Calculation of doses of solid drug forms
- Conversion between units
- Calculation of doses of liquids

▶ INTRODUCTION

In many settings, drugs are dispensed in unit-dose systems (see Figure 4.3, page 52). However, even in these settings, there are situations that require dosage calculations such as stat doses, liquid preparations, and prn doses. Therefore, accurate calculation is extremely important. This module describes how to calculate solid and liquid forms for oral administration, and it provides practice exercises so you can develop an accurate and consistent approach. Clinical practice will further develop these skills.

CRITICAL POINT

Each time that you administer a medication, check that you follow the classic "five rights of medication administration." These are as follows:

Right drug: Read the medication order and the label. Use medications only from legibly labelled containers.[1]

Right dose: Calculate and validate. Remember to use one approach to calculate the dose and another method to validate.[2]

Right route: Read the medication order and the label.

Right time: Read the medication order and check that it is not outdated. Read the chart to confirm the last time the medication was administered. Read the label to check the expiry date.

Right patient: Read the medication administration record (MAR). Check the patient's identification (ID) band. Ask the patient to state his or her name.

(Continued)

---

[1] It is beyond the scope of this book to teach pharmacotherapeutics. In addition to checking the order and the label, you are also expected to have a knowledge of pharmacology, drug–food interactions, drug–drug interactions, and patient factors such as drug-related allergy.

[2] Some agencies require that drug calculations (e.g., doses for children) be checked by a second person. Always check policies in the clinical setting.

CRITICAL POINT *(Continued)*

In addition, there are three other "rights":

Right technique: Use aseptic procedures and know injection sites, for example.

Right approach: Explain the medication to the patient and family, and calm a child before an injection, for example.

Right recording: Accurate charting after administration according to policy/records in the setting is crucial.

▶ DEFINITIONS

Please note that this book uses the following terms:

Dose: a portion of any therapeutic agent (drug) to be administered at one time (e.g., 325 mg of acetaminophen)

Dosage: a system of doses; that is, the dose and the frequency of administration (e.g., acetaminophen 325 mg PO q4h)

Strength or concentration: the available supply on hand stated as the amount of drug per tablet/capsule or the amount of drug dissolved in solution (e.g., 325 mg/tab; 10 mg/mL)

▶ USE OF A CALCULATOR

Many practitioners use one method to calculate a drug dose (e.g., proportion) and then use a calculator to verify the answer. This practice can safeguard against human error.

Calculation of Decimals

To perform operations involving decimal numbers on a calculator, enter the numerals from left to right and press the decimal point after the last whole number.

Examples: Enter 2.64

Enter ❷

Enter decimal •

Enter ❻

Enter ❹

Thus ❷ • ❻ ❹

To enter 164.25

Enter ❶ ❻ ❹ • ❷ ❺

Example: Using a calculator, convert 5'4" to centimetres.

Write out the proportion statements:

> 1 in. = 2.54 cm
> 1 ft. = 12 in.

Convert 5'4" to inches:

> Enter ❺ × ❶❷ = 60; then add ❹.
>
> Thus 5'4" equals 64 inches.

Use proportion (extremes = means) to solve:

> 1 in.:2.54 cm = 64 in.:x cm
>
> $1x = 2.54 \times 64$

Enter ❷ • ❺❹ × ❻❹ = 162.56 cm

Calculation of Fractions

To perform operations involving fractions on a calculator, first convert the fraction to a decimal number. Recall the relationship between the numerator and the denominator. The fraction $\frac{1}{2}$ is the same as stating 1 of 2.

Example: You are to give $\frac{1}{2}$ of a 0.25-mg tab. How many milligrams will the patient receive?

Using a calculator, convert the fraction to a decimal:

> Enter ❶ ÷ ❷ = 0.5

Multiply: $0.5 \times 0.25 = 0.125$

The patient will receive 0.125 mg.

CRITICAL POINT

Always write out the proportion statement, including the units of measurement, before using a calculator. Doing the operation "in your head" will increase the risk of error.

▶ CALCULATION OF DOSES OF SOLID DRUG FORMS

The oral route is the most common route for drug administration. Oral drug forms include solid forms, such as tablets and capsules, and liquids, such as elixirs, syrups, and suspensions. Tablets or capsules contain a specific weight of a drug, commonly expressed in milligrams or grams. Liquid forms contain a specific amount of medication in a solvent (e.g., water or alcohol).

There are four methods for calculating solid drug forms.

Method A: ratio and proportion: extremes = means
Method B: ratio and proportion: cross multiplication
Method C: formula statement
Method D: problem-solving approaches

CRITICAL POINT

You should decide which method you prefer and then use the same method consistently. It is recommended that you use one method to do the calculation and use another method to validate the answer. This will enhance accuracy.

Let's use the following order to illustrate each method:

Order: rofecoxib 50 mg PO daily
Supply: rofecoxib (Vioxx) 25-mg tablets

Method A: Extremes = Means

Known ratio: 25 mg/1 tab

Unknown ratio: 50 mg/x tab

Write the proportion statement; check that units are consistent across the equation:

$$\overbrace{25 \text{ mg}:1 \text{ tab}}^{\text{means}} = 50 \text{ mg}:x \text{ tab}$$
extremes

Solve for x: $25x = 50$

$$x = (50 \div 25) = 2$$

Give 2 tablets.

Method B: Cross Multiplication

Known ratio: $\dfrac{25 \text{ mg}}{1 \text{ tab}}$

Unknown ratio: $\dfrac{50 \text{ mg}}{x \text{ tab}}$

Write the proportion statement; check that units are consistent across the equation:

$$\frac{25}{1} = \frac{50}{x}$$

Solve for x: $\dfrac{25}{1} \diagdown \dfrac{50}{x}$

$$25x = 50$$

$$x = (50 \div 25) = 2$$

Give 2 tablets.

CRITICAL POINT

When using proportion equations, be certain to check that the units of measurement (e.g., milligrams, tablets, millilitres) are consistent across the equation.

Solve the example using a formula. Several nursing books use a variety of "formula statements" for calculation. These formula statements instruct that the dose is divided by the available supply.

Method C: Formula Statement

$$\frac{\text{Dose (medication order)}}{\text{Supply (available strength/concentration)}} \times \text{Vehicle} = \text{Amount to administer}$$

For oral tablets or capsules, the dose is the medication order, the supply is the strength of the tablet/capsule, and the vehicle is one tablet or capsule. The calculation shown below is for the order of rofecoxib.

Example:

$$\frac{50 \text{ mg (medication order)}}{25 \text{ mg (strength per tablet)}} \times 1 \text{ tab (vehicle)} = 2 \text{ tabs (amount to administer)}$$

CRITICAL POINT

Relying on a formula presents some disadvantages. You might forget or misuse the formula. Also, you cannot validate the answer with the formula; you must use the proportion equation. Therefore, the author does not encourage the formula method.

Method D: Problem-Solving Approaches

You may have your own method of problem solving. It is acceptable to use this method, provided that you are consistent and that you use one of the other methods to validate the answer. See Appendix D for an example of the problem-solving approach.

Study the following example and then proceed to Exercise 5.1 to practise using one method to calculate and another to validate the answer.

Study the label in Figure 5.1. The label states that the bottle contains 120 caplets and that each caplet contains 325 mg of acetaminophen. Calculate the number of caplets needed to give a dose of 650 mg. Calculate using cross multiplication, and validate using a formula statement.

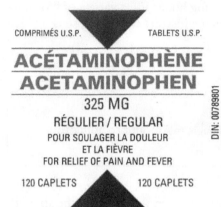

COMPRIMÉS U.S.P.   TABLETS U.S.P.

ACÉTAMINOPHÈNE
ACETAMINOPHEN

325 MG

RÉGULIER / REGULAR

POUR SOULAGER LA DOULEUR
ET LA FIÈVRE
FOR RELIEF OF PAIN AND FEVER

120 CAPLETS   120 CAPLETS

DIN: 00789801

Il est peu probable que l'acétaminophène provoque des dérangements d'estomac ou de l'irritation gastrique. Il agit rapidement pour soulager temporairement les maux de tête, les douleurs musculaires, la douleur associée aux crampes menstruelles et la fièvre.

POSOLOGIE ORALE POUR ADULTES: Prendre 1 ou 2 caplets et répéter à toutes les 4 heures au besoin. La dose quotidienne maximale est de 12 caplets ou tel que recommandé par le médecin. Il est dangereux de dépasser la dose maximale quotidienne recommandée sans consulter un médecin. Consulter un médecin si la situation exige l'usage continu pendant plus de 5 jours. LIRE LE FEUILLET D'INFORMATION.

MISE EN GARDE: Ce contenant renferme suffisamment de médicaments pour être gravement nocif à un enfant.

CONSERVER CE MÉDICAMENT HORS DE LA PORTÉE DES ENFANTS.

BOUCHON SCELLÉ POUR VOTRE PROTECTION.

Acetaminophen is unlikely to cause stomach upset or gastric irritation and acts quickly to provide temporary relief from headaches, muscular aches, pain caused by menstrual cramps and fever.

ADULT ORAL DOSE: Take 1 or 2 caplets, repeat every 4 hours if necessary. The maximum daily dose is 12 caplets or as recommended by a physician. It is hazardous to exceed the maximum recommended dose unless advised by a physician. Consult physician if the underlying condition requires continued use for more than 5 days. READ DIRECTION CIRCULAR.

CAUTION: This package contains enough drug to seriously harm a child.

KEEP OUT OF REACH OF CHILDREN.

CAP SEALED FOR YOUR PROTECTION.

Trianon   LABORATOIRES TRIANON INC. BLAINVILLE (QUÉBEC) J7C 3V4

FIGURE 5.1

Trianon Laboratories Inc., Blainville, Quebec.

Example:

Known ratio: 1 cap = 325 mg

Unknown ratio: x caps = 650 mg

$$\frac{325 \text{ mg}}{1 \text{ cap}} = \frac{650 \text{ mg}}{x \text{ caps}}$$

$$325x = 650$$

$$x = (650 \div 325) = 2 \text{ caps}$$

Validation: $\dfrac{\text{Dose}}{\text{Supply}} \times \text{Vehicle} = \text{Amount to administer}$

$$\frac{650 \text{ mg}}{325 \text{ mg}} \times 1 \text{ cap} = 2 \text{ caps}$$

The above example is relatively simple, and you may be tempted to "see" the answer — that 650 is 2×325. Some drug doses are not so simple, as is shown in the following exercises.

CRITICAL POINT

Throughout this book, you will be asked to calculate a specific dose by using the available supply (strength or concentration) of a drug product. You must always state the answer in full; that is, including *tablets* or *millilitres*, for example.

Some calculations look easy, and you can see the answer immediately. Always check your answer intuitively: does it make sense? However, you should also develop a thorough and careful approach to calculations; develop the habit of validating your answer. Calculate — then validate.

▶ EXERCISE 5.1

Answer questions 1 to 5 without referring to the above text. Calculate using one method, and validate using another method. Correct your answers by using the answer guide starting on page 192. (Value: 2 marks each: 1 for a correct answer, 1 for validation)

1. Order: 0.125 mg PO daily. Available supply: 0.25-mg tablets.

2. Order: 0.15 mg PO daily. Available supply: 0.05-mg tablets.

3. Order: 0.015 g PO bid. Available supply: 0.005-g tablets.

4. Order: 0.1 mcg PO daily. Available supply: 0.05-mcg tablets.

5. Order: 12.5 mg PO daily. Available supply: 50-mg scored (quadrisect) tablets.

Your Score: /10   =   %

▶ EXERCISE 5.2

Complete the following exercise. Calculate the dose using one method, then validate using another method. State the answer in full (include tablets or caplets). Correct your answers by using the answer guide starting on page 192. (Value: 3 marks each: 1 for a correct calculation, 1 for validation, and 1 for including the correct unit in the answer)

1. Order: benazepril hydrochloride 40 mg per day in 2 divided doses
   Supply: Study the labels in Figure 5.2. State the product strength that you are using.
   Calculate:
   Validate:

2. Order: Voltaren 75 mg PO
   Supply: Study the labels in Figure 5.3. State the product strength that you are using.
   Calculate:
   Validate:

3351-11-00A

Adult Dose: Initially, 10 mg once a day. The usual maintenance dose is 20 mg daily. Do not exceed 40 mg per day. Product monograph supplied on request. Protect from heat (i.e. store at 15-30°C) and humidity.

Novartis Pharmaceuticals Canada Inc.
Novartis Pharma Canada inc.
Dorval (Québec) H9S 1A9

℗**Lotensin® 10 mg**
benazepril hydrochloride tablets
comprimés de chlorhydrate de bénazépril

DIN 00885843   1755

Ϣ NOVARTIS

Angiotensin Converting Enzyme Inhibitor
Inhibiteur de l'enzyme de conversion de l'angiotensine
100 tablets/comprimés

Posologie pour adulte :
Débuter avec 10 mg une fois par jour. La dose d'entretien habituelle est de 20 mg par jour. Ne pas dépasser 40 mg par jour. Monographie fournie sur demande. Protéger de la chaleur (c.-à-d. conserver entre 15 et 30°C) et de l'humidité.

3373-11-00A

Adult Dose: Initially, 10 mg once a day. The usual maintenance dose is 20 mg daily. Do not exceed 40 mg per day. Product monograph supplied on request. Protect from heat (i.e. store at 15-30°C) and humidity.

Novartis Pharmaceuticals Canada Inc.
Novartis Pharma Canada inc.
Dorval (Québec) H9S 1A9

℗**Lotensin® 20 mg**
benazepril hydrochloride tablets
comprimés de chlorhydrate de bénazépril

DIN 00885851   1740

Ϣ NOVARTIS

Angiotensin Converting Enzyme Inhibitor
Inhibiteur de l'enzyme de conversion de l'angiotensine
100 tablets/comprimés

Posologie pour adulte :
Débuter avec 10 mg une fois par jour. La dose d'entretien habituelle est de 20 mg par jour. Ne pas dépasser 40 mg par jour. Monographie fournie sur demande. Protéger de la chaleur (c.-à-d. conserver entre 15 et 30°C) et de l'humidité.

FIGURE 5.2
Novartis Pharmaceuticals Canada Inc., Dorval, Quebec.

3356-11-00A

Usual adult dosage: *Osteoarthritis:* Initial and maintenance dose is 25 mg three times daily. *Rheumatoid arthritis:* Initially: 25-50 mg three times daily depending on the severity of the condition. For maintenance: 25 mg three times daily or the minimum amount to provide continuous control of symptoms. Maximum daily dose is 150 mg. Tablets should be swallowed whole, with food. Not recommended for use in patients under 16 years of age. Product monograph supplied on request. Protect from heat and humidity. **PHARMACIST: Dispense with the PATIENT INFORMATION LEAFLET provided to you.**

Novartis Pharmaceuticals Canada Inc.
Novartis Pharma Canada inc.
Dorval (Québec) H9S 1A9

℗**Voltaren® 25 mg**
diclofenac sodium tablets
comprimés de diclofénac sodique

DIN 00514004   2551

Ϣ NOVARTIS

Anti-inflammatory analgesic agent
Agent anti-inflammatoire – analgésique

100 enteric-coated tablets
100 comprimés entéro-solubles

Posologie habituelle pour adulte :
Ostéoarthrite: Dose d'attaque et d'entretien habituelle : 25 mg trois fois par jour. *Arthrite rhumatoïde:* Dose d'attaque : 25 à 50 mg trois fois par jour selon la gravité du cas. Dose d'entretien : 25 mg trois fois par jour ou administrer la dose minimale qui produit un contrôle continu des symptômes. La dose maximale quotidienne est de 150 mg. Les comprimés doivent être avalés entiers, avec de la nourriture. Non recommandé chez les patients de moins de 16 ans. Monographie fournie sur demande. Protéger de la chaleur et de l'humidité. **PHARMACIEN: Remettre avec le feuillet INFORMATION POUR LE PATIENT qu'on vous a fourni.**

Usual adult dosage: *Osteoarthritis:* Initial and maintenance dose is 25 mg three times daily. *Rheumatoid arthritis:* Initially: 25-50 mg three times daily depending on the severity of the condition. For maintenance: 25 mg three times daily or the minimum amount to provide continuous control of symptoms. Maximum daily dose is 150 mg. Tablets should be swallowed whole, with food. Not recommended for use in patients under 16 years of age. Product monograph supplied on request. Protect from heat and humidity. **PHARMACIST: Dispense with the PATIENT INFORMATION LEAFLET provided to you.**

℗**Voltaren® 50 mg**
diclofenac sodium tablets
Anti-inflammatory analgesic agent
Agent anti-inflammatoire – analgésique

Ϣ NOVARTIS

100 enteric-coated tablets
100 comprimés entéro-solubles

DIN 00514012   2561

Posologie habituelle pour adulte : *Ostéoarthrite:* Dose d'attaque et d'entretien habituelle : 25 mg trois fois par jour. *Arthrite rhumatoïde:* Dose d'attaque : 25 à 50 mg trois fois par jour selon la gravité du cas. Dose d'entretien : 25 mg trois fois par jour ou administrer la dose minimale qui produit un contrôle continu des symptômes. La dose maximale quotidienne est de 150 mg. Les comprimés doivent être avalés entiers, avec de la nourriture.

Non recommandé chez les patients de moins de 16 ans. Monographie fournie sur demande. Protéger de la chaleur et de l'humidité. **PHARMACIEN: Distribuer avec le feuillet INFORMATION POUR LE PATIENT qu'on vous a fourni.**

Novartis Pharmaceuticals Canada Inc.
Novartis Pharma Canada inc.
Dorval (Québec) H9R 4P5
3021-11-97A

FIGURE 5.3
Novartis Pharmaceuticals Canada Inc., Dorval, Quebec.

3. Order: baclofen 15 mg PO tid
   Supply: Study the labels in Figure 5.4. Note that both products are scored tablets.
   State the product strength that you are using.
   Calculate:
   Validate:

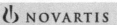

Usual adult dosage: Titration begins with 5 mg 3 times a day for 3 days, followed by increases to 10, 15, and 20 mg 3 times a day at 3-day intervals. Maximum dose should not exceed 80 mg daily (20 mg 4 times a day). Not recommended in children. If benefits are not evident after a trial period, the medication should be withdrawn slowly. Product monograph supplied on request. Protect from heat and humidity.
Novartis Pharmaceuticals Canada Inc.
Novartis Pharma Canada inc.
Dorval (Québec) H9S 1A9

ⓅLioresal®10mg
baclofen tablets USP
comprimés de baclofène USP

DIN 00455881   1635

Ⓤ NOVARTIS

Muscle relaxant, antispastic
Relaxant musculaire, antispastique
100 tablets
100 comprimés

Posologie habituelle pour adulte : Instituer le traitement avec 5 mg 3 fois par jour pour 3 jours; augmenter la dose à 10, 15, et 20 mg 3 fois par jour à 3 jours d'intervalle. La dose maximale ne devrait pas dépasser 80 mg par jour (20 mg 4 fois parw jour). L'emploi chez l'enfant n'est pas conseillé. Si après une période d'essai la réponse n'est pas satisfaisante, *le sevrage devrait se faire lentement.* Monographie fournie sur demande. Protéger de la chaleur et de l'humidité.

Usual Adult Dosage: Titration begins with 5 mg 3 times a day for 3 days, followed by increases to 10, 15 and 20 mg 3 times a day at 3-day intervals. Maximum dose should not exceed 80 mg daily (20 mg 4 times a day). Not recommended in children. If benefits are not evident after a trial period, the medication should be withdrawn slowly. Product monograph supplied on request. Protect from heat and humidity.
Novartis Pharmaceuticals Canada Inc.
Novartis Pharma Canada inc.
Dorval (Québec) H9S 1A9

ⓅLioresal®D.S. 20mg
baclofen tablets USP
comprimés de baclofène USP

DIN 00636576   1640

Ⓤ NOVARTIS

Muscle relaxant, antispastic
Relaxant musculaire, antispastique
100 tablets
100 comprimés

Posologie habituelle pour adulte : Instituer le traitement avec 5 mg 3 fois par jour pour 3 jours; augmenter la dose à 10, 15 et 20 mg 3 fois par jour à 3 jours d'intervalle. La dose maximale ne devrait pas dépasser 80 mg par jour (20 mg 4 fois par jour). L'emploi chez l'enfant n'est pas conseillé. Si après une période d'essai la réponse n'est pas satisfaisante, *le sevrage devrait se faire lentement.* Monographie fournie sur demande. Protéger de la chaleur et de l'humidité.

FIGURE 5.4
Novartis Pharmaceuticals Canada Inc., Dorval, Quebec.

4. Order: clomipramine 125 mg PO daily
   Supply: Study the labels in Figure 5.5. State the product strength that you are using.
   Calculate:
   Validate:

5. Order: Anafranil 75 mg PO daily
   Supply: Study the labels in Figure 5.5. State the product strength that you are using.
   Calculate:
   Validate:

6. Order: theophylline 450 mg PO pc
   Supply: theophylline (Theo-Dur) 300-mg scored tabs
   Calculate:
   Validate:

3344-11-00A

Adult dosage: Depression and Obsessive Compulsive Disorder (OCD): Initially 25 mg daily, increase gradually by 25 mg up to 150-200 mg. Severely depressed patients, up to 300 mg daily. Severe cases of OCD, up to 250 mg daily. **Children and adolescents: For OCD treatment only:** Initially 25 mg daily, increase gradually up to a maximum of 200 mg daily. Maintain at lowest effective dose. Product monograph supplied on request. Protect from heat (store between 2 and 30°C).

Novartis Pharmaceuticals Canada Inc.
Novartis Pharma Canada Inc.
Dorval (Québec) H9S 1A9

℞ **Anafranil® 25mg**
clomipramine hydrochloride tablets
comprimés de chlorhydrate de clomipramine

DIN 00324019   1122

ᛦ NOVARTIS

Antidepressant, Antiobsessional
Antidépresseur, Anti-obsessionnel

100 tablets
100 comprimés

Posologie pour adultes: dépression et troubles obsessionnels compulsifs (TOC): Au début, 25 mg par jour; augmenter graduellement par paliers de 25 mg jusqu'à 150 à 200 mg. Dépression sévère, jusqu'à 300 mg par jour. Troubles obsessionnels compulsifs sévères, jusqu'à 250 mg par jour. **Enfants et adolescents en traitement de TOC seulement:** Au début, 25 mg par jour; augmenter graduellement jusqu'à un maximum de 200 mg par jour. Maintenir à la plus faible dose efficace. Monographie fournie sur demande. Protéger de la chaleur (conserver entre 2 et 30°C).

3345-11-00A

Adult dosage: Depression and Obsessive Compulsive Disorder (OCD): Initially 25 mg daily, increase gradually by 25 mg up to 150-200 mg. Severely depressed patients, up to 300 mg daily. Severe cases of OCD, up to 250 mg daily. **Children and adolescents: For OCD treatment only:** Initially 25 mg daily; increase gradually up to a maximum of 200 mg daily. Maintain at lowest effective dose. Product monograph supplied on request. Protect from heat (store between 2 and 30°C).

Novartis Pharmaceuticals Canada Inc.
Novartis Pharma Canada Inc.
Dorval (Québec) H9S 1A9

℞ **Anafranil® 50mg**
clomipramine hydrochloride tablets
comprimés de chlorhydrate de clomipramine

DIN 00402591   1126

ᛦ NOVARTIS

Antidepressant, Antiobsessional
Antidépresseur, Anti-obsessionnel

100 tablets
100 comprimés

Posologie pour adultes: dépression et troubles obsessionnels compulsifs (TOC): Au début, 25 mg par jour; augmenter graduellement par paliers de 25 mg jusqu'à 150 à 200 mg. Dépression sévère, jusqu'à 300 mg par jour. Troubles obsessionnels compulsifs sévères, jusqu'à 250 mg par jour. **Enfants et adolescents en traitement de TOC seulement:** Au début, 25 mg par jour; augmenter graduellement jusqu'à un maximum de 200 mg par jour. Maintenir à la plus faible dose efficace. Monographie fournie sur demande. Protéger de la chaleur (conserver entre 2 et 30°C).

FIGURE 5.5
Novartis Pharmaceuticals Canada Inc., Dorval, Quebec.

7. Order: bromocriptine mesylate 5 mg PO daily
   Supply: bromocriptine mesylate (Parlodel) 2.5-mg tablets
   Calculate:
   Validate:

8. Order: nadolol 40 mg PO hs
   Supply: nadolol (Corgard) 80-mg scored tablets
   Calculate:
   Validate:

9. Order: meperidine 75 mg PO for pain
   Supply: meperidine (Demerol) 50-mg scored tablets
   Calculate:
   Validate:

10. Order: hydrochlorothiazide 100 mg PO daily
    Supply: hydrochlorothiazide (HydroDiuril) 50-mg tablets
    Calculate:
    Validate:

11. Order: atorvastatin calcium (Lipitor) 30 mg PO
    Supply: Two bottles of tablets labelled 10 mg and 20 mg. Be sure to state which strength you are using and how many tablets to administer.
    Calculate:
    Validate:

12. Order: digoxin 0.125 mg PO daily
    Supply: digoxin (Lanoxin) 0.25-mg scored tablets
    Calculate:
    Validate:

13. Order: levothyroxine sodium 0.1 mg PO daily
    Supply: levothyroxine sodium (Eltroxin) 0.05-mg tablets
    Calculate:
    Validate:

14. Order: captopril 6.25 mg PO tid
    Supply: quadrisect scored tablets 25 mg
    Calculate:
    Validate:

15. Order: Aspirin 650 mg PO
    Supply: Aspirin 325-mg tablets
    Calculate:
    Validate:

Your Score:	/45	=	%

▶ CONVERSION BETWEEN UNITS

Sometimes, the dose and the supply on hand are in different units of measurement. In these situations, *you must convert and express the dose and the available strength/concentration in the same units.* Recall the conversions you made in Module 3. Study the following example and then proceed to the exercise for practice.

Example: The order is for a dose of 1.5 g. The supply on hand is 500-mg capsules. State the dose in milligrams.

Convert: 1.5 g = 1500 mg (recall: 1 g = 1000 mg)

Calculate: $\dfrac{500 \text{ mg}}{1 \text{ cap}} = \dfrac{1500 \text{ mg}}{x \text{ caps}}$

Note that the units are the same on both sides of the equation: cancel the units and solve for x.

$$500x = 1500$$

$$x = (1500 \div 500) = 3$$

Give 3 caps.

Validation: 500 mg:1 cap = 1500 mg:3 caps

$$500 \times 3 = 1 \times 1500$$

$$1500 = 1500$$

▶ EXERCISE 5.3

Answer the questions without referring to the above text. Correct your answers by using the answer guide starting on page 192. (Value: 2 marks each: 1 for a correct conversion, 1 for a correct calculation)

1. Order: 0.125 mg PO daily
   Supply: 125-mcg tablets
   Give: _____

2. Order: 0.5 g PO qid
   Supply: 250-mg capsules
   Give: _____

3. Order: 0.25 mg PO tid
   Supply: 250-mcg tablets
   Give: _____

4. Order: 0.45 g PO q8h
   Supply: 150-mg capsules
   Give: _____

5. Order: 1 g stat
   Supply: 250-mg tablets
   Give: _____

Your Score:	/10	=	%

▶ CALCULATION OF DOSES OF LIQUIDS

Medications may be administered orally in suspensions and solutions. You should learn the following definitions:

Solution: one or more drugs dissolved in a liquid.

Suspension: fine particles of a drug suspended in a liquid base. A suspension appears cloudy and must be shaken well before using. Examples include emulsions, magmas, and gels.

Elixir: an aromatic sweetened solution containing a dissolved medication. Elixirs contain various percentages of alcohol.

Calculation of liquid forms should be done using proportion (either extremes = means or cross multiplication, as you prefer).

NOTE: Although some references use a formula statement, the author does not recommend this method as it has a greater risk of error in calculation.

CRITICAL POINT

Oral liquid medications are often poured into a 1 fl. oz. measuring cup. When measuring liquid, it is important to view the curve of the liquid, called the meniscus, at eye level. You should read the bottom of the curve, as illustrated in Figure 5.6.

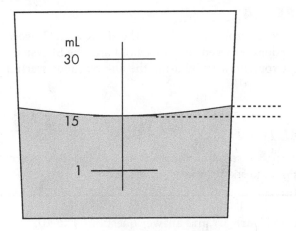

FIGURE 5.6 Reading a meniscus. A meniscus is caused by the surface tension of a solution against container walls. The surface tension causes the formation of a concave or hollowed curvature on the solution surface. Read the level at the lowest point of the concave curve.

Review the sample problem and then proceed to Exercise 5.4 for practice in calculating oral liquid doses.

Problem: The order is for thioridazine hydrochloride 60 mg PO prn, and the available concentration is thioridazine hydrochloride 25 mg/5 mL.

Method A: Extremes = Means

Known ratio: 25 mg/5 mL

Unknown ratio: 60 mg/x mL

Check that units are consistent across the equation.

$$25 \text{ mg}:5 \text{ mL} = 60 \text{ mg}:x \text{ mL}$$

$$25x = 300$$

$$x = (300 \div 25) = 12$$

Give 12 mL to provide a dose of 60 mg.

Validation: $\dfrac{25 \text{ mg}}{5 \text{ mL}} = \dfrac{60 \text{ mg}}{12 \text{ mL}}$

$$25 \times 12 = 5 \times 60$$

$$300 = 300$$

Method B: Cross Multiplication

Known ratio: $\dfrac{25 \text{ mg}}{5 \text{ mL}}$

Unknown ratio: $\dfrac{60 \text{ mg}}{x \text{ mL}}$

Check that units are consistent across the equation.

$$\dfrac{25 \text{ mg}}{5 \text{ mL}} \diagup\!\!\!\!\times\!\!\!\!\diagdown \dfrac{60 \text{ mg}}{x \text{ mL}}$$

$$25x = 300$$

$$x = (300 \div 25) = 12$$

Give 12 mL to provide a dose of 60 mg.

Validation: 25 mg:5 mL = 60 mg:12 mL

$$25 \times 12 = 5 \times 60$$

$$300 = 300$$

► EXERCISE 5.4

Complete the exercise without referring to the above text. However, if you have difficulty doing the conversions between the household and the SI systems, review Table 3.4 on page 41. Correct your answers by using the answer guide starting on page 192. (Value: 1 mark each)

CRITICAL POINT

Dosage errors often result from carelessness. Whenever you calculate a dosage, check the answer to see if it seems reasonable.

Study the labels in Figure 5.7 and answer questions 1 to 10.

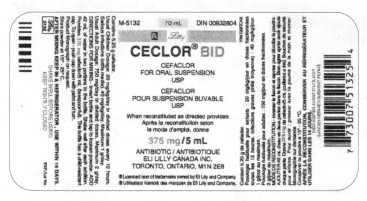

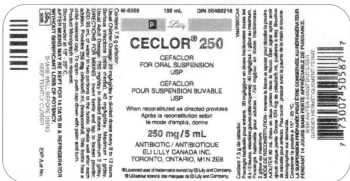

FIGURE 5.7

© 2001, Eli Lilly Canada, Inc. Reproduced by permission. Eli Lilly Canada, Inc., Scarborough, Ontario. All rights reserved.

1. What is the product brand name?

2. What is the product generic name?

3. State the concentration of each oral suspension.

4. Outline the directions for reconstitution for each product. How much water should be added?

5. For Ceclor 250, calculate a dose of 125 mg.

6. For Ceclor 250, state how many milligrams are contained in 1 tsp.

7. If an adult took 2 tbsp. of the Ceclor 250 suspension, how much drug would be received? Does this exceed the maximum daily dose?

8. The order is Ceclor BID 750 mg PO daily in 2 divided doses. Calculate each dose.

9. The label for Ceclor BID states that the maximum adult dose is 2 g/day. How many millilitres would contain the maximum dose? Round to the nearest whole number.

10. Read both labels. Which product contains the greatest total amount of drug?

Your Score:	/10	=	%

▶ EXERCISE 5.5

This exercise is designed to give you an opportunity to practise reading labels. No score is given for this exercise, but check your answers against comments provided in the answer guide starting on page 192. Study all the labels in this module and locate the following information:

1. What is the usual adult dose? Are dosages given for children?

2. Are maximum daily doses given?

3. Who is the manufacturer?

4. What is the brand name? What is the generic name?

5. Are storage instructions provided?

6. Are other instructions provided?

▶ EXERCISE 5.6

This activity is designed to help you develop a consistent and accurate approach to setting up the problem before you calculate the answer. Each of the following problems and calculations has an error. Find the error and determine the correct calculation. Correct your answers by using the answer guide starting on page 192. (Value: 2 marks each: 1 for finding the error, 1 for the correct answer)

1. Order: phenobarbital 0.3 g PO

   Supply: phenobarbital 100-mg tablets

   Calculate: 0.3 g = 3000 mg

   $$\frac{100 \text{ mg}}{1 \text{ tab}} = \frac{3000 \text{ mg}}{x \text{ tabs}}$$

   $100x = 3000$

   $x = 30$

   Give 30 tabs? Does this make sense? *Find the error.*

2. Order: warfarin 5 mg PO

   Supply: warfarin 2.5-mg tablets

   Calculate: ("see" the answer) 2.5 ÷ 5 = 0.5 tab

   Give 0.5 tab? *What went wrong?*

3. Order: 2500 mg
   Supply: 1-g tablets
   Calculate: 1:1 tab = 2500:x tabs
              $x = 2500$

   Give 2500 tabs? Obviously, there is a serious error here; you cannot possibly give 2500 tabs. *What went wrong?*

4. Order: 30 mg of an elixir
   Supply: elixir labelled 15 mg/5 mL
   Calculate: 5:15 = 30:x
              $5x = 450$
              $x = 90$

   Give 90 mL? *What went wrong?*

5. Order: digoxin 0.125 mg
   Supply: digoxin 0.25-mg tablets
   Calculate: ("see" the answer) 0.125 ÷ 0.25 = 5 tabs

   Give 5 tabs? Too often, the nurse might "see" the answer without carefully writing out the problem. This error actually does occur in the clinical setting (and it is very serious). *Find the error.*

Your Score:	/10	=	%

▶ CASE STUDY

Complete the case study questions without referring to the above text. Correct your answers by using the answer guide starting on page 192.

Mr. B., a 79-year-old man, is admitted to an acute care hospital with congestive heart failure. Medication orders include the following:

Lasix 80 mg PO today then 40 mg daily
digoxin 0.375 mg today only
digoxin 0.25 mg PO starting tomorrow
levothyroxine sodium 0.075 mg daily

Study the "medication cupboard" in Figure 5.8 and answer questions 1 to 15.

1. State the generic and trade name of each product. (Value: 6 marks)
2. State the available strengths for each of the following drugs: Lanoxin, Lasix, Synthroid, Eltroxin. (Value: 12 marks)

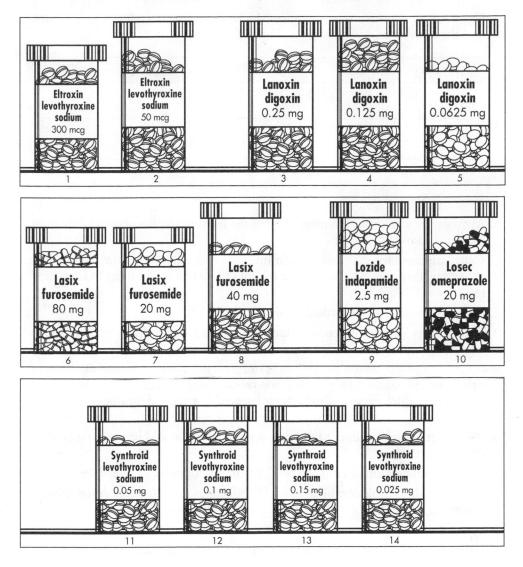

FIGURE 5.8 Medication cupboard

3. Calculate all doses for today for Mr. B. State which product you are using and the number of tablets to give. (Value: 6 marks)

Product	Number of Tablets to Give

4. Calculate all doses for tomorrow for Mr. B. State which product you are using and the number of tablets to give. (Value: 6 marks)

Product	Number of Tablets to Give

5. Arrange the strengths of Synthroid from the greatest (highest dose) to the least. (Value: 1 mark)

6. Calculate doses for the morning administration of omeprazole for the following 3 days: day 1: 60 mg PO A.M.; day 2: 80 mg PO A.M.; day 3: 60 mg PO A.M. and 40 mg PO hs. (Value: 3 marks)

7. Calculate how to give Lozide 2.5 mg PO. (Value: 1 mark)

8. The order is for levothyroxine sodium 0.3 mg. Which product will you use, and why? (Value: 1 mark)

9. If 0.05 mg of levothyroxine sodium is ordered, calculate all possible choices of products and amounts to give. Assume tabs are *not* scored; whole tabs must be used. State which products and strengths would be most desirable to use. (Value: 4 marks)

10. If 1 tablet of each product of digoxin is given, what would be the total dosage? (Value: 1 mark)

11. State the strength of all Lanoxin products in micrograms. (Value: 3 marks)

12. Calculate all possible combinations of products to give 80 mg of furosemide. Example: Give 1 tab of 80 mg. (Value: 3 marks)

13. Calculate an order of Synthroid 100 mcg PO. (Value: 1 mark)

14. Calculate an order of digoxin 125 mcg PO. (Value: 1 mark)

15. Calculate an order of Losec 20 mg PO. (Value: 1 mark)

Your Score:	/50	=	%

▶ POST-TEST

Instructions

1. Write the post-test without referring to any resources.
2. Correct the post-test by using the answer guide starting on page 192. (Value: 1 mark each)
3. Be careful to include all units with the answer (e.g., caplets, millilitres, tablets).
4. Validate all answers.

Order: ampicillin 500 mg PO bid
Supply: 250-mg caps of ampicillin. Answer questions 1 and 2.
  1. Calculate the number of caps for each dose.
  2. Calculate the number of caps required for one day's supply.

Order: cephalexin 1 g PO q6h
Supply: cephalexin 500-mg tabs. Answer questions 3 and 4.
  3. Calculate the number of tabs for each dose.
  4. Calculate the number of tabs required for one week's supply.

Order: digoxin 125 mcg PO qam
Supply: digoxin 0.125-mg tabs. Answer question 5.
  5. Calculate the number of tabs for one dose.

Order: penicillin G potassium 1 000 000 units PO qid
Supply: penicillin G potassium tablets labelled 500 000 units. Answer question 6.
  6. Calculate the number of tabs for each dose.

Order: sulfasalazine 1 g PO qid
Supply: sulfasalazine 500-mg tabs. Answer question 7.
  7. Calculate the number of tabs for each dose.

Order: glyburide 1.25 mg PO
Supply: glyburide 2.5-mg scored tablets. Answer question 8.
  8. Calculate the dose to administer.

The patient is to receive 35 mg of an elixir. The bottle label reads 15 mg/5 mL. Answer questions 9 and 10.
  9. If 2 mL was given, what dose did the patient receive?
  10. How many millilitres should the patient receive for one dose? (Round to a whole number.)

The drug order is for 500 mg q6h. The drug label reads 250 mg/5 mL. Answer questions 11 and 12.
  11. How much drug should be given for one dose?
  12. If the bottle contains 150 mL, how many doses can be given from this supply?

The patient has been taking Aspirin for 24 hours and took 2 tablets every 4 hours. Each tablet is 325 mg. Answer questions 13 and 14.
  13. How many milligrams has the patient had in total?
  14. How many grams?

Order: levothyroxine 150 mcg PO
Supply: levothyroxine tablets labelled 0.15 mg. Answer question 15.
  15. Calculate the number of tabs per dose.

Order: Tylenol No. 3 Elixir equivalent to 2 tabs q4h. Note: Each tablet contains 320 mg of acetaminophen and 30 mg of codeine. Acetaminophen elixir contains 160 mg/5 mL of acetaminophen. Codeine syrup contains 5 mg/mL of codeine. Answer questions 16 and 17.
  16. Calculate how much elixir to administer.
  17. Calculate how much syrup to give per dose.

  18. The order is for morphine sustained release 175 mg PO bid. The available drug supply is MS Contin 15-mg, 30-mg, 60-mg, 100-mg, and 200-mg tablets. (Note: Sustained-release tablets must not be cut.) Select the product strength and calculate the amount to give.

19. The order is for digoxin 0.1875 mg PO daily. The available drug supply is digoxin 0.25-mg, 0.125-mg, and 0.0625-mg tablets. Select the product strength and calculate the amount to give.

Order: KCl 30 mEq PO bid
Supply: (a) bottle label reads potassium chloride (K-10) liquid 20 mEq in 15 mL; (b) tablets labelled 750 mg = 10 mEq/tab. Answer questions 20 and 21. Do not round your answers.

20. Calculate the dose for administration in liquid form. (Note: The liquid form of this medication is always diluted in water, orange juice, or tomato juice.)

21. Calculate the dose for administration of tablets.

22. The order is for nystatin suspension 500 000 units swish and swallow. The available drug supply is labelled nystatin 100 000 units/mL. Calculate the amount to give.

Read the following labels for penicillin V potassium and answer questions 23 to 26.

Penicillin concentration	Potassium (mEq)	Potassium (mg)
250-mg (400 000-unit) tablets	0.72	28.06
500-mg (800 000-unit) tablets	1.44	56.12
oral solution:		
250 mg (400 000 units)/5 mL	0.72	28.06

23. If a patient received 2 tablets of 250 mg, how many units of penicillin were given?

24. If a patient received 4 mL of the oral solution, how many milligrams of penicillin were given?

25. How many milligrams of potassium are equal to 1 mEq of potassium?

26. If a patient received 10 mL of oral solution, how many mEq of potassium were received?

Order: Lotensin 15 mg PO daily
Supply: Study the labels in Figure 5.2 (page 74) and Figure 5.9. Answer question 27.

3350-11-00A

Adult Dose: Initially, 10 mg once a day. The usual maintenance dose is 20 mg daily. Do not exceed 40 mg per day. Product monograph supplied on request.
Protect from heat (i.e. store at 15-30°C) and humidity.

Novartis Pharmaceuticals Canada Inc.
Novartis Pharma Canada inc.
Dorval (Québec) H9S 1A9

℗ **Lotensin® 5mg**
benazepril hydrochloride tablets
comprimés de chlorhydrate de bénazépril

DIN 00885835   1750

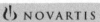
Ⓤ **NOVARTIS**

Angiotensin Converting Enzyme Inhibitor
Inhibiteur de l'enzyme de conversion de l'angiotensine
100 tablets/comprimés

Posologie pour adulte :
Débuter avec 10 mg une fois par jour. La dose d'entretien habituelle est de 20 mg par jour. Ne pas dépasser 40 mg par jour. Monographie fournie sur demande.
Protéger de la chaleur (c.-à-d. conserver entre 15 et 30°C) et de l'humidité.

FIGURE 5.9
Novartis Pharmaceuticals Canada Inc., Dorval, Quebec.

27. State the product strength that you are using and calculate the amount to give.

Study the label in Figure 5.10 and answer questions 28 to 31.

Adult dose for rheumatoid arthritis and osteoarthritis: Once a maintenance dosage of 75 mg per day has been established with Voltaren® enteric coated tablets, a once-daily dose of Voltaren® SR 75 mg may be substituted, taken morning or evening. Patients on a maintenance dose of 150 mg per day may be changed to a twice daily dose of one Voltaren® SR 75 mg tablet taken morning and evening. Tablets should be swallowed whole with liquid, preferably at mealtime. Maximum daily dose for Voltaren® in any dosage form is 150 mg. Not recommended for use in patients under 16 years of age. Product monograph supplied on request. Store at room temperature and protect from humidity. **PHARMACIST: Dispense with the PATIENT INFORMATION LEAFLET provided to you.**

ᴾ**Voltaren®SR 75**mg
diclofénac sodium
diclofénac sodique

Anti-inflammatory analgesic agent
Agent anti-inflammatoire –
analgésique

ᴜ NOVARTIS

100 slow release tablets
100 comprimés à libération
lente
DIN 00782459   2540

0 63601 02540 7

Posologie pour adulte dans l'arthrite rhumatoïde et l'ostéo-arthrite : Lorsque la dose d'entretien a été établie à 75 mg par jour avec les comprimés entéro-solubles de Voltaren®, on peut substituer le comprimé Voltaren® SR 75 mg administré une fois par jour, le matin ou le soir. Chez les patients qui prennent une dose d'entretien de 150 mg par jour, on peut la remplacer par une dose biquotidienne de Voltaren® SR 75 mg, soit un comprimé pris le matin et un le soir. Avaler les comprimés entiers avec du liquide, de préférence au repas. La dose maximale de Voltaren® sous

toutes ses formes est de 150 mg par jour. Non recommandé chez les patients de moins de 16 ans. Monographie fournie sur demande. Garder à la température ambiante et à l'abri de l'humidité. **PHARMACIEN: Distribuer avec le feuillet INFORMATION POUR LE PATIENT qu'on vous a fourni.**

Novartis Pharmaceuticals Canada Inc.
Novartis Pharma Canada inc.
Dorval (Québec) H9R 4P5
3019-11-98B

FIGURE 5.10
Novartis Pharmaceuticals Canada Inc., Dorval, Quebec.

28. State the brand name.
29. State the trade name.
30. State the maximum daily dose.
31. When can the daily dose be administered?

Order: Voltaren 75 mg PO
Supply: Study the labels in Figure 5.3 (page 74) and Figure 5.10. Answer question 32.
32. State the product strength that you are using and calculate two preferable options to give.

Order: Lioresal 5 mg PO tid
Supply: Study the labels in Figure 5.4 (page 75). Note that both products are scored tablets. Answer question 33.
33. State the product strength that you are using and calculate the amount to give.

Study the labels in Figure 5.5 (page 76) and answer questions 34 to 36.
Order: clomipramine 175 mg PO daily
34. State the product strength that you are using and calculate the amount to give.

Order: Anafranil 300 mg PO daily
35. State the product strength that you are using and calculate the amount to give.
36. If a patient overdosed and took all the tablets in the bottle labelled Anafranil 25 mg, how many grams would the patient have received?

Study the label in Figure 5.9. Answer questions 37 to 40.
37. What is the brand name?
38. What is the generic name?
39. Calculate the initial dose.
40. Calculate the usual maintenance dose.

Your Score:	/40	=	%

Did you achieve 100%?

YES — Proceed to Module 6.

NO — Analyze your areas of weakness and review this module; then rewrite the post-test. If your score is still less than 100%, please seek remedial assistance.

Calculation of Parenteral Medication Doses

▶ **MODULE TOPICS**

- Reading of calibrated medication equipment
- Calculation of parenteral medication doses
- Reconstitution of powdered medication

▶ **INTRODUCTION**

Administration of medications by the parenteral route (SC, IM, or IV) requires greater precision than administration by the oral route. Whereas you might measure a teaspoon (approximately 5 mL), you will calculate and give parenteral doses such as 0.4 mL and 1.25 mL. Drugs for parenteral administration must be in liquid form and are supplied in the following containers:

1. Disposable syringes used for single doses (e.g., epinephrine [EpiPen])

2. Ampules for single-dose use (e.g., meperidine 50 mg/mL)

3. Vials for single- or multi-dose use

4. Vials containing powder or crystals that must be mixed with a diluent (e.g., many antibiotics)

CRITICAL POINT

It is safe clinical practice to always calculate parenteral doses on paper and to validate your work. In some clinical settings, it is a requirement to double-check the dose with a colleague. Know the policies of each setting.

▶ **READING OF CALIBRATED MEDICATION EQUIPMENT**

Before studying the calculation of liquid medications for parenteral administration, you should be familiar with the calibration of syringes. This module does not acquaint you with the procedure of injections. Examine the figures only to become familiar with the calibration of each type of syringe (see Figure 6.1).

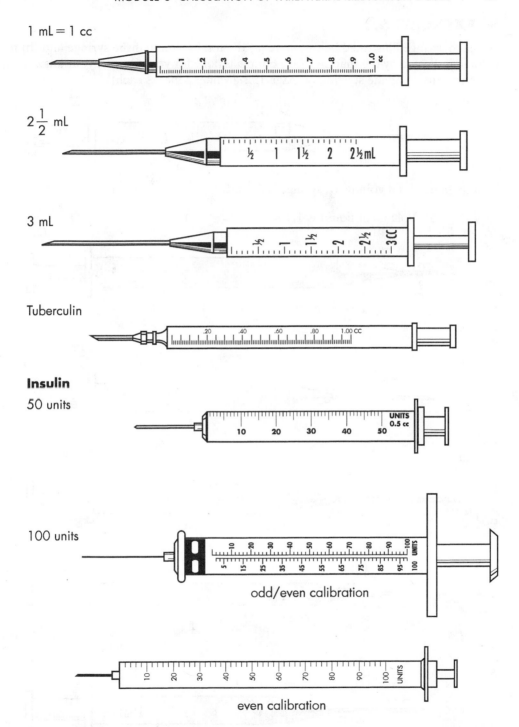

FIGURE 6.1 Syringes

▶ **EXERCISE 6.1**

For each syringe illustrated below, state (a) the total volume of the syringe and (b) the volume indicated by the shading. An example is done for you. Correct your answers by using the answer guide starting on page 192. (Value: 2 marks each)

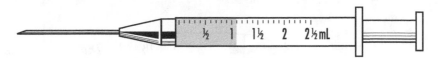

Example: a. Total volume of syringe is $2\frac{1}{2}$ mL.

b. Volume of liquid is 1.1 mL.

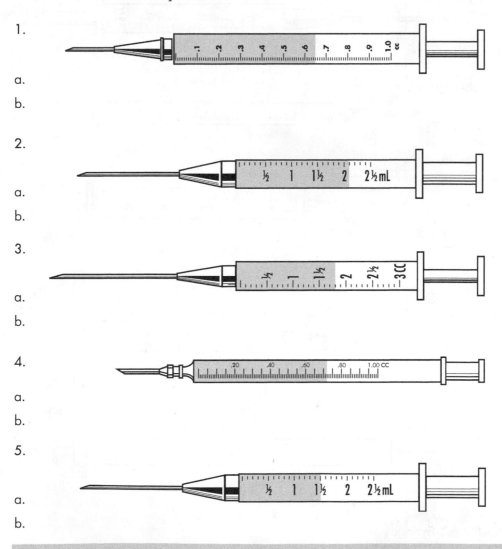

1.

a.

b.

2.

a.

b.

3.

a.

b.

4.

a.

b.

5.

a.

b.

Your Score: /10 = %

▶ CALCULATION OF PARENTERAL MEDICATION DOSES

Once again, there are different approaches to calculating doses of parenteral liquid medications. You should use the same method consistently and always validate your answer.

Method A: ratio and proportion: extremes = means
Method B: ratio and proportion: cross multiplication
Method C: formula statement
Method D: problem-solving approaches

Problem: Give 75 mg IM using a 2-mL ampule labelled "50 mg/mL."

Method A: Extremes = Means

Known ratio: 50 mg in 1 mL

Unknown ratio: 75 mg in x mL

$$50{:}1 = 75{:}x$$

$$50x = 75$$

$$x = (75 \div 50) = 1.5$$

Give 1.5 mL.

Validation: $\dfrac{50}{1} = \dfrac{75}{1.5}$

$$75 = 75$$

Method B: Cross Multiplication

Known ratio: 50 mg/1 mL

Unknown ratio: 75 mg/x mL

$$\frac{50}{1} \diagdown\hspace{-0.9em}\times \frac{75}{x}$$

$$50x = 75$$

$$x = (75 \div 50) - 1.5$$

Give 1.5 mL.

Validation: $50{:}1 = 75{:}1.5$

$$50 \times 1.5 = 1 \times 75$$

$$75 = 75$$

Method C: Formula Statement

$$\frac{\text{Dose (medication order)}}{\text{Supply (available strength/concentration)}} \times \text{Vehicle} = \text{Amount to administer}$$

$$\frac{75\ \text{mg}}{50\ \text{mg}} \times 1\ \text{mL} = x\ \text{mL}$$

$$x = 1.5$$

Give 1.5 mL.

Always include the units to ensure that you have set up the formula correctly. There are disadvantages to using the formula method. First, you may forget the formula or you may insert the values into the formula incorrectly. Second, it is difficult to validate the answer; ratio and proportion must be used for validation.

Check your answer "intuitively." For example, a 2-mL ampule contains 100 mg of drug (50 mg per mL); to give 75 mg, you have calculated 1.5 mL. Does your calculation seem right?

Method D: Problem-Solving Approaches

You may have your own method of problem solving. It is acceptable to use this method, provided that you are consistent and that you use one of the other methods to validate the answer. See Appendix D for an example of the problem-solving approach.

CRITICAL POINT

Always write decimal numbers according to the rules. For example, write 1.6 mL not 1.60 mL.

▶ **EXERCISE 6.2**

Complete the following exercise without referring to the above text. Ensure that the appropriate units are part of your answer (e.g., milligrams, millilitres). Round decimal numbers to the nearest hundredth. Correct your answers by using the answer guide starting on page 192. (Questions 1 to 6 value: 2 marks each: 1 for calculation, 1 for correct unit)

1. The order is for heparin 7500 units SC. You have a 5-mL vial of heparin labelled "10 000 units/mL." Determine the correct volume to administer.

2. The label on a 2-mL ampule indicates 50 mg/mL. How many milligrams are contained in 1.5 mL?

3. The vial label states "250 mg ampicillin per mL." Calculate 400 mg IM.

4. Your patient has an order for meperidine (Demerol) 75 mg IM. The 2-mL ampule is labelled "50 mg/mL." How many millilitres should the patient receive?

5. The drug label states "100 mg/mL." Calculate an 80-mg dose.

6. The antibiotic label states "400 000 units/mL." If 1 mg = 1600 units, calculate how many millilitres are required to deliver a dose of 200 mg.

For each of the following questions, *shade* in the accompanying syringe to indicate the correct volume. (Value: 2 marks each: 1 for calculation, 1 for correct shading)

7. Ordered: heparin 5000 units SC
   Supply: heparin 10 000 units/mL

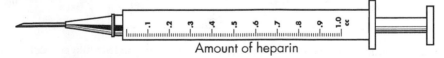

Amount of heparin

8. Ordered: morphine 12 mg IM
   Supply: morphine 15 mg/mL

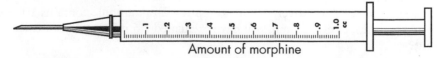

Amount of morphine

9. Ordered: dimenhydrinate (Gravol) 30 mg IM prn
   Supply: dimenhydrinate 50 mg/mL

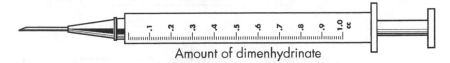

Amount of dimenhydrinate

10. An analgesic is ordered: 75 mg IM stat. On hand is a 2-mL ampule with a dosage concentration of 50 mg/mL. Calculate the volume to administer.

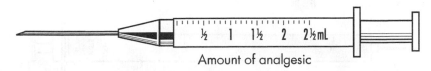

Amount of analgesic

Your Score: /20 = %

▶ **EXERCISE 6.3**

Read the volume of medication in each of the syringes below. Correct your answers by using the answer guide starting on page 192. (Value: 1 mark each)

1.

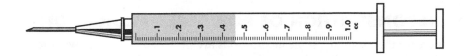

2.

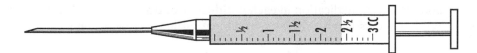

3.

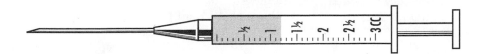

4.

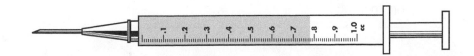

5.

6.

7.

8.

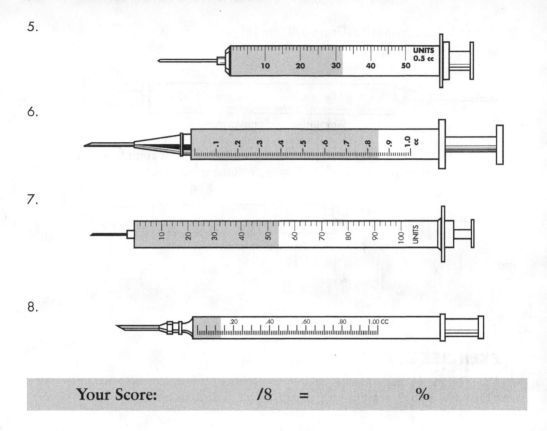

Your Score: /8   =   %

▶ RECONSTITUTION OF POWDERED MEDICATION

To increase their stability, some medications are prepared in a dry-powder form and must be diluted with a sterile solvent before administration. For example, many antibiotics must be reconstituted with sterile water. Refer to Table 6.1, which illustrates a dilution table on a multidose vial. Note that adding 46 mL of sterile diluent yields a solution with 200 000 IU of medication in each millilitre. Contrast this concentration with the solution that results when only 6 mL of diluent, usually sterile water, are added.

TABLE 6.1 Reconstitution of a Powdered Drug

Potency Required (IU per mL)	Sterile Aqueous Diluent to Add (mL)
200 000	46
250 000	36
750 000	9.3
1 000 000	6

> **CRITICAL POINT**
>
> When a certain volume of liquid is added to a powdered drug in a vial, the resulting product will usually be of a greater volume. For example, adding 9.3 mL of fluid may result in a final volume in the vial of 10 mL. The powdered drug occupies some volume.

To prepare a liquid from a powder form,

1. Read the directions on the label or package insert.
2. Select the diluent (the label will state at least one of):
   - Sterile water for injection
   - Bacteriostatic water (which has a preservative)
   - Normal saline for injection
3. Decide what concentration to prepare based on the required dose and route of administration.
4. Inject air into the vial of diluent to create positive pressure, and withdraw the desired volume of diluent.
5. Inject the diluent into the vial of powdered drug. Shake well to produce a homogeneous mixture.

   NOTE: Some products should not be shaken. Read the instructions with each drug.
6. Calculate and withdraw the correct volume for the required dose.
7. Date and initial the vial; indicate the volume of diluent added.
8. Store the vial according to the directions.

Study the following example and Figure 6.2, then proceed to Exercise 6.4.

Example: A vial of penicillin G potassium contains 5 million units of drug. Package instructions specify "sterile water for injection."

Directions are as follows:

Volume of Diluent to Be Added (mL)	Approximate Available Volume (mL)	Approximate Concentrations (Potency) (IU/mL)
3	5	1 000 000
8	10	500 000
18	20	250 000

To give a dose of 250 000 IU, for example, you would add 18 mL of sterile water for injection, shake well to mix evenly, and withdraw 1 mL.

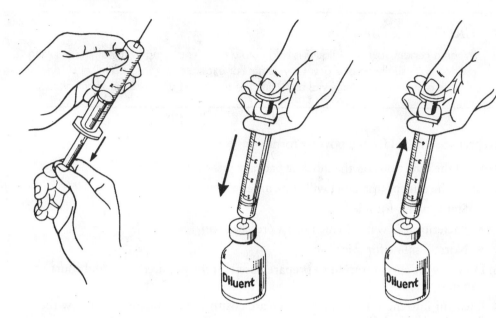

1. Draw back plunger.

2. Inject air into diluent.

3. Withdraw desired volume of diluent.

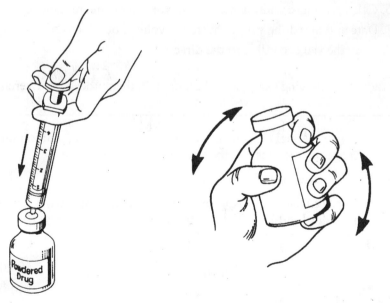

4. Inject diluent into vial of powdered medication.

5. Mix drug thoroughly.

FIGURE 6.2 Reconstitution of a powdered drug form

NOTE: In the example on page 95, 17 mL remain in the vial for future use. It is the responsibility of the person who reconstitutes the vial to label it with the date and the concentration of the contents, and to initial the vial. Although reconstituted drugs may be stored at room temperature, they remain stable for longer periods in the refrigerator. Practise reading labels in the clinical setting to become familiar with this technique.

CRITICAL POINT

Always indicate the concentration on the vial, after you add diluent. For example,

9.6 mL	100 000 units/mL
4.6 mL	200 000 units/mL
1.6 mL	500 000 units/mL

CRITICAL POINT

When reconstituting powdered medications, ensure that the drug is dissolved thoroughly. Shake the vial well, and allow it to sit until any foam has settled. Examine for any precipitate or particulate matter; if this occurs, attempt to dissolve the drug or discard the vial and contents. If discolouration occurs, consult drug literature; if abnormal, discard the vial and contents.

▶ EXERCISE 6.4

Study the following label and answer questions 1 to 8. Round all answers to the nearest tenth. Correct your answers by using the answer guide starting on page 192. (Value: 1 mark each)

Potency Required (IU per mL)	Sterile Aqueous Diluent to Add (mL)
200 000	46
250 000	36
750 000	9.3
1 000 000	6

1. The order is for 750 000 units IM q4h. How much diluent would you add to yield a solution with a concentration of 750 000 units/mL?

2. The medication has been mixed by another nurse and the vial is signed, dated, and marked to indicate that 9.3 mL of sterile diluent was added. How much would be required to administer a dose of 1 million units?

You add 46 mL of sterile diluent to the powdered drug. For each of the following orders, indicate the correct volume to administer:

3. 750 000 units

4. 400 000 units

5. 250 000 units

You add 36 mL of sterile diluent to the powdered drug. For each of the following volumes, indicate the amount of drug (in units):

6. 1 mL

7. 0.8 mL

8. 1.4 mL

Study the label in Figure 6.3 and answer questions 9 to 12.

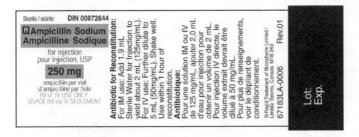

FIGURE 6.3

Novopharm Limited, Toronto, Ontario.

9. State the volume and type of diluent to be added for IM use.

10. How long is the reconstituted solution stable?

11. Calculate the volume to administer 200 mg.

12. What routes can be used with this product?

Study the label in Figure 6.4 and answer questions 13 to 17.

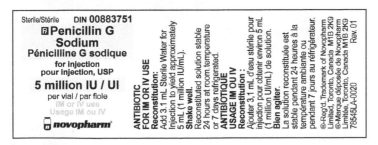

FIGURE 6.4

Novopharm Limited, Toronto, Ontario.

13. State the name of the drug.

14. State the volume and type of diluent for IM use.

15. State the resulting concentration.

16. How long is the reconstituted solution stable?

17. Calculate the volume to give a dose of 1 million units.

18. A penicillin vial is labelled 200 000 units/mL. The order is 80 000 units IM. Determine the correct volume to give.

19. The order is for perphenazine 3.5 mg IM stat. The ampule is labelled 5 mg/mL. Determine the correct volume to administer.

20. From a container of hydrocortisone 100 mg/2 mL, determine the correct dose for 75 mg IM daily.

Your Score: /20   =   %

▶ EXERCISE 6.5

This exercise is designed to help you practise recognizing errors. For each of the following situations, indicate whether the calculation is correct. If incorrect, state the correct answer. Correct your answers by using the answer guide starting on page 192. (Value: 2 marks each)

1. The order is for 2500 units SC bid and the available strength is 10 000 units/mL. Your coworker has drawn up 2.5 mL. *Is this correct?*

2. The order is dimenhydrinate 50 mg IM stat. The available concentration is in an ampule labelled "50 mg/mL." *Is 1 ampule the correct amount to administer?*

3. Fluphenazine decanoate 12.5 mg IM is ordered. A 10-mL vial is labelled "fluphenazine decanoate 25 mg/mL." *Is the correct volume 2 mL?*

4. A coworker asks you to double-check the drug dosage. The order is for 4300 units, the label states 1000 units/mL, and the syringe indicates 4 mL has been drawn up. *Correct?*

5. An ampule is labelled 60 mg/2 mL. The order is for a stat dose of 45 mg. You calculate 1.5 mL. Validate. *Correct?*

Your Score: /10   =   %

CRITICAL POINT

Dosage calculation in the clinical setting requires several steps. You should approach each situation in the same way to develop consistency; this will lead to confidence and competence. Note that the labels on different products vary; therefore, you must always read carefully. To review, the steps are as follows:

1. Read the medication order.
2. Locate the medication.
3. Read the label carefully (three times).
4. Calculate the dosage and validate your answer.

NOTE: Always use the same method to calculate (choose the method that you prefer), and then use another method to validate the answer.

▶ EXERCISE 6.6

This exercise provides an additional opportunity to practise reading medication labels carefully. Complete the following exercise without referring to the above text. Correct your answers by using the answer guide starting on page 192. (Value: 1 mark each)

Study the label in Figure 6.5 and answer questions 1 to 5.

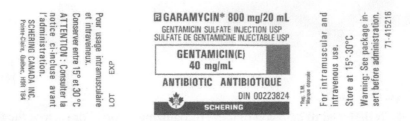

FIGURE 6.5
Schering Canada Inc., Pointe-Claire, Quebec.

1. State the trade name.
2. State the generic name.
3. How much drug is contained in the vial?
4. Calculate the volume for an order of gentamicin 65 mg IM. Round to the nearest tenth.
5. By what routes can this drug be given?

Study the labels in Figure 6.6 and answer questions 6 to 10.

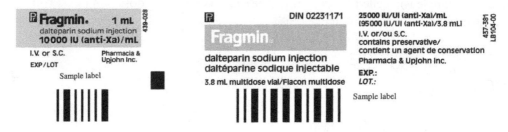

FIGURE 6.6
Pharmacia Canada Inc., Mississauga, Ontario.

6. State the volume in each of the products.
7. State the concentration of the drug in each product, expressed in IU/mL.
8. State the routes of administration.
9. Using the 3.8-mL multidose vial, calculate the volume for an order of 2500 IU sc 1 h preoperative. Calculate using one method and validate using another method.
10. The labels in Figure 6.6 illustrate the importance of reading labels very carefully before withdrawing a drug. Which product has the greatest concentration? If you withdrew 1 mL of the product labelled 25 000 IU/mL instead of 1 mL of the product labelled 10 000 IU/mL, what is the degree of error?

Study the label in Figure 6.7 and answer questions 11 to 15.

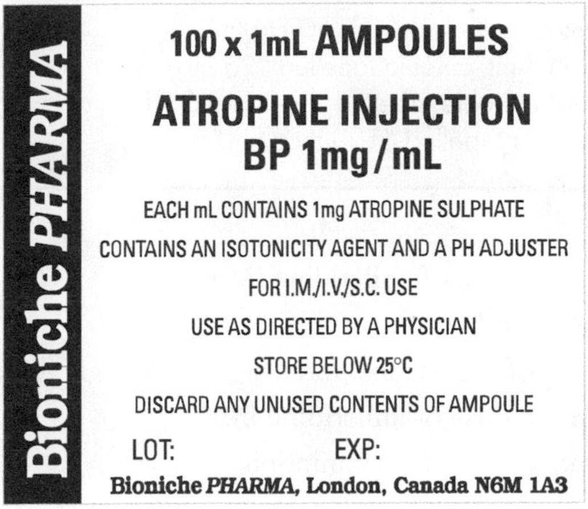

100 x 1mL AMPOULES

**ATROPINE INJECTION
BP 1mg/mL**

EACH mL CONTAINS 1mg ATROPINE SULPHATE

CONTAINS AN ISOTONICITY AGENT AND A PH ADJUSTER

FOR I.M./I.V./S.C. USE

USE AS DIRECTED BY A PHYSICIAN

STORE BELOW 25°C

DISCARD ANY UNUSED CONTENTS OF AMPOULE

LOT: EXP:

Bioniche PHARMA, London, Canada N6M 1A3

Bioniche PHARMA

FIGURE 6.7
Bioniche Pharma Group, London, Ontario.

11. State the concentration of the drug.
12. State all the components in the drug product.
13. State the recommended routes of administration.
14. Calculate the volume to give for an order of atropine 0.6 mg sc.
15. Validate the answer in question 14.

| Your Score: | /15 | = | % |

▶ **CASE STUDY**

This exercise provides additional practice through a simulated clinical situation. Answer the questions without referring to the above text. Round all answers to the nearest tenth. Correct your answers by using the answer guide starting on page 192. (Value: 2 marks each: 1 for calculation, 1 for validating your answer using another method)

Mrs. E.G., a 94-year-old woman, is admitted to acute care for investigation of abdominal pain. She has no known allergies. Medication orders include the following:

dimenhydrinate 50 mg IM q3–4h prn for nausea
anileridine phosphate 15–25 mg IM q4–6h prn for pain
acetaminophen liquid 325–650 mg PO q4h prn for pain
cyanocobalamin injections 100 mcg IM daily × 3 days

(Continued)

(Continued)
Supply:
dimenhydrinate 1-mL ampule labelled "50 mg/mL"
anileridine phosphate 1-mL ampule labelled "25 mg/mL"
acetaminophen liquid in bottle labelled "160 mg/5 mL"
cyanocobalamin ampule labelled "100 mcg/mL"

1. Calculate the minimum dose of anileridine IM stat.
2. Calculate dimenhydrinate IM stat.
3. Calculate today's dose of cyanocobalamin.
4. Calculate the maximum dose of anileridine IM.
5. Calculate the minimum dose of acetaminophen.

Your Score: /10 = %

▶ OPTIONAL ACTIVITY

NOTE: Recall from Module 4 that drug labels are not standardized. Reading labels requires attention and experience. You should always read the drug label three times: once as you take it from the shelf, drawer, or cupboard; again as you compare the label with the order; and again after you have calculated the dosage.

During a clinical experience, ask a nurse to show you the variety of drug products and labels of powdered-drug products. Select a few vials and/or boxes or package inserts and find the following:

* Recommended diluent and resulting concentration after reconstitution
* Stability at room temperature and when refrigerated
* Total weight of drug in the vial
* Route of administration

Practise some calculations; look at the possible concentrations that can be prepared, and calculate various doses.

▶ POST-TEST

Instructions

1. Write the post-test without referring to any resources.
2. Round decimal numbers to the nearest hundredth.
3. Correct the post-test by using the answer guide starting on page 192. (Value: 1 mark each)

Study the label in Figure 6.8 and answer questions 1 to 4. Imagine the label indicates that 3.5 mL of diluent was added at 13:00 h.

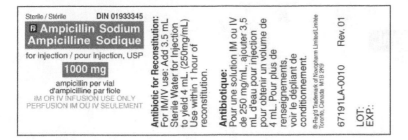

FIGURE 6.8
Novopharm Limited, Toronto, Ontario.

1. State the concentration of the solution.
2. Calculate 250 mg IM.
3. State the hour when the drug becomes outdated.
4. State the total amount of drug in the vial.
5. The order is perphenazine 3.5 mg IM stat. The ampule is labelled "5 mg/mL." Determine the correct volume to administer.
6. From a supply of hydrocortisone 100 mg/2 mL, determine the correct volume for 75 mg IM daily.
7. The order is for meperidine 75 mg IM prn. The ampule is labelled "meperidine 100 mg/mL." Determine the correct volume to administer.
8. Study the label in Figure 6.9 and calculate the volume for a dose of morphine 7.5 mg sc stat.
9. Study the label in Figure 6.9 and state the amount of drug in a volume of 0.53 mL.

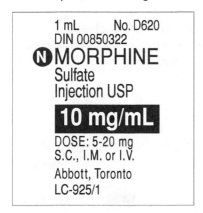

FIGURE 6.9
Reprinted with permission of Abbott Laboratories, Limited, Montreal, Quebec.

10. Study the label in Figure 6.10 and calculate the volume for a dose of phenobarbital 25 mg IM.
11. Study the label in Figure 6.10 and state the volume of drug in a volume of 0.78 mL.

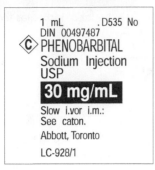

1 mL   . D535 No
DIN 00497487
Ⓒ PHENOBARBITAL
Sodium Injection
USP
30 mg/mL
Slow i.vor i.m.:
See caton.
Abbott, Toronto
LC-928/1

FIGURE 6.10
Reprinted with permission of Abbott Laboratories, Limited, Montreal, Quebec.

Two concentrations of naloxone are in supply: product A is a 1-mL ampule labelled "0.4 mg/mL"; product B is a 2-mL ampule labelled "0.02 mg/mL." Answer questions 12 to 16 based on this information.

12. Which naloxone product has the greatest concentration?

13. The recommended adult dose is 100 mcg to 200 mcg every 2 to 3 minutes until adequate ventilation and alertness are achieved. The order is to give 200 mcg IV stat. Calculate the volume to give, and state which product you are using.

14. The recommended dose for an infant is 10 mcg/kg. The infant weighs 8.5 kg. Calculate the volume to give, and state which product you are using. Round to the nearest hundredth.

15. If you withdrew 0.5 mL of product A but intended to withdraw the same volume of product B, what is the error?

16. The naloxone product labelled "0.4 mg/mL" is used; 1 mL is given sc and is repeated in 2 minutes and again in 3 minutes. What is the total dose received?

17. The order is for phytonadione (vitamin K) 1 mg sc stat. The ampule is labelled "10 mg/mL." Calculate the volume to give.

18. The order is for RhoGAM (Rho(D) immune globulin) 300 mcg IM. The label reads "1500 IU = 300 mcg." The drug is accompanied by a special diluent. Dilute the powder with 1.25 mL of the diluent to result in a final solution with a concentration of 1200 IU/mL. Calculate the volume to give.

19. Order: diphenhydramine 20 mg sc stat
    Supply: diphenhydramine 50 mg/mL
    Calculate the volume to give.

20. Order: dimenhydrinate 30 mg IM stat
    Supply: dimenhydrinate 50 mg/5 mL
    Calculate the volume to give.

Your Score: /20   =   %

Did you achieve 100%?

YES — Proceed to Module 7.

NO — Analyze your areas of weakness and review this module; then rewrite the post-test. If your score is still less than 100%, please seek remedial assistance.

Intravenous Administration

▶ MODULE TOPICS

- Calculation of rate of flow of intravenous infusions
- Interpretation of abbreviations related to intravenous therapy
- Continuous intravenous medication administration
- Preparation and calculation of intravenous medications for intermittent administration

▶ INTRODUCTION

Today, in most settings (including the home), many drugs are given by the intravenous route. Absorption of the drug is fast and reliable, the route usually causes less pain than the intramuscular route, and modern devices such as heparin and saline locks allow the individual to have freedom of movement. However, the intravenous route also has risks: the drugs are not retrievable after administration, and the preparation and administration of the drug are more complex. This module encourages you to develop confidence in the procedure for preparing the drug and calculating for intravenous administration.

▶ CALCULATION OF RATE OF FLOW OF INTRAVENOUS INFUSIONS

All intravenous fluids and medications must be administered precisely. The desired rate of flow must be calculated accurately and observed frequently during IV therapy.

The volume and type of IV fluid are ordered by the physician. The safe rate of intravenous administration is determined by many factors, including the following:

1. Age: infants and the elderly tolerate less fluid
2. Cardiovascular status
3. Site of the infusion
4. Nature of the infusion; for example, irritating fluids or medications must be infused slowly to allow for adequate hemodilution

Intravenous fluids are administered either by electronic controller devices or by gravity drip. This module focuses on clinical situations involving a gravity drip. Figures 7.1A and 7.1B illustrate IV administration equipment.

To calculate the rate of flow for a gravity drip, you must know the following:

1. The volume of IV fluid ordered
2. The time for infusion
3. The IV tubing calibration, also called the drop factor (i.e., the calibration of the administration set in drops per millilitre)

Macrodrip or standard sets have a drop factor of 10, 15, or 20 drops/mL. In contrast, a minidrip produces a very small drop and 60 drops/mL (see Figure 7.2). The calibration is printed on the IV package. The macrodrip or standard set is used most commonly. However, in some situations, the infusion rate is to be very slow; if an electronic controller device is not available, a minidrip set can be used. The minidrip set is commonly used in veterinary medicine.

The physician's order for IV fluids is often written in millilitres per hour (e.g., 125 mL/h). Orders may also be written as 1000 mL/8h or 1 L q8h.

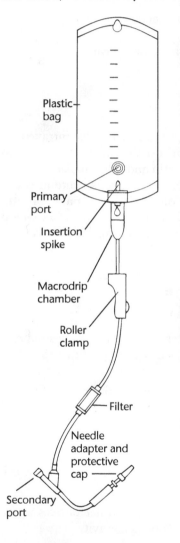

Plastic bag

Primary port

Insertion spike

Macrodrip chamber

Roller clamp

Filter

Needle adapter and protective cap

Secondary port

Système InterLink® System

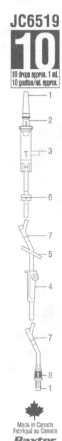

JC6519

10

10 drops approx. 1 mL
10 gouttes/mL approx.

To open package, tear vertically at notch
Pour ouvrir, déchirer à l'encoche

Continu-Flo® Solution Set
Dispositif Continu-Flo® pour solutés

2 Injection Sites, Male Luer Lock Adapter
2 Sites d'injection, Adaptateur "Luer Lock" Mâle

81" (2.1 m) long
Fluid path is sterile, nonpyrogenic.
Cautions: Do not use if tip protectors (1) are not in place.
Do not place on sterile field.

La canalisation est stérile et apyrogène.
Mise en garde: Ne pas utiliser si les protecteurs (1) sont détachés.
Ne pas déposer sur un champ stérile.

Directions: Use aseptic technique.
Close regulating clamp (4). Insert spike (2) into solution container. Fill drip chamber (3) to fill line. Open regulating clamp (4). If flow does not start, squeeze plastic container. Invert and tap check valve (6) to purge air during priming. Prime set, purge air. Close regulating clamp (4) until roller meets bottom of frame. Attach male Luer adapter (8) to Interlink® cannula or vascular access device using a firm push and twist motion and then engage the Luer lock collar to prevent accidental disconnection.
To properly set flow, always close regulating clamp (4) until roller meets bottom of frame, then reopen to establish flow rate. Repeat procedure if adjusting clamp from fully open position.

Cautions:
Do not allow air to be trapped in set.
Puncturing set components may cause air embolism.
If needle must be used, insert small gauge needle into perimeter of septum (7).
Do not disconnect administration set, syringe or other component from cannula while cannula is still connected to Interlink® injection site.
Single use only. Do not resterilize.

Notes:
This set contains DEHP.
Swab septum of injection site (7) with antiseptic prior to access.
Access Interlink® injection site (7) (identified by a colored ring) with Interlink® cannula. See cannula directions.
This product does not contain natural rubber latex.
For secondary medication administration, use upper Y-injection site only. See directions for use with secondary medication set.
To stop flow without disturbing regulating device (4), close slide clamp (5).
Replace set per CDC guidelines.
Major plastic material in contact with fluids: Polyvinyl Chloride.

Mode d'emploi: Utiliser une technique aseptique.
Fermer la pince régulatrice (4). Insérer le perfuseur (2) dans le contenant de soluté. Remplir la chambre de débit (3) jusqu'à la ligne de remplissage. Ouvrir la pince régulatrice (4). Si le liquide ne s'écoule pas, presser le contenant de plastique. Inverser et tapoter la valve d'arrêt (6) afin d'expulser l'air. Remplir le dispositif, expulser l'air. Fermer la pince régulatrice (4) en plaçant la roulette fermement au bas de la pince. Fixer l'adaptateur Luer mâle (8) à une canule Interlink® ou au dispositif d'accès vasculaire en exerçant une pression et en tournant. Engager ensuite le collet à verrouillage Luer pour empêcher une déconnexion accidentelle.
Afin de régler correctement l'écoulement, toujours fermer la pince régulatrice (4) en plaçant la roulette fermement au bas de la pince, puis ouvrir de nouveau pour régler le débit. Répéter la procédure pour ajuster la pince lorsqu'elle est en position complètement ouverte.

Mise en garde:
Il ne doit pas y avoir d'air dans la canalisation.
Toute perforation des composantes du dispositif peut provoquer une embolie gazeuse.
Si une aiguille doit être utilisée, insérer une aiguille de petit calibre dans le périmètre de la membrane (7).
Ne pas détacher un dispositif d'administration, seringue ou autre composante de la canule lorsque la canule est reliée au site d'injection Interlink®.
Usage unique seulement. Ne pas restériliser.

Notes:
Ce dispositif contient du "DEHP".
Nettoyer la membrane du site d'injection (7) avec un antiseptique avant son utilisation.
Utiliser la canule Interlink® dans le site d'injection Interlink® (7) (identifié par un anneau de couleur autour de la membrane). Consulter les directives de la canule.
Ce produit ne contient pas de caoutchouc naturel vulcanisé.
Pour administrer tout médicament secondaire, utiliser le site d'injection supérieur seulement. Voir le mode d'emploi pour utiliser le dispositif secondaire.
Pour interrompre l'écoulement sans modifier le régulateur de débit (4), utiliser la pince à glissière (5).
Remplacer le dispositif selon les directives du CDC.
La principale matière plastique en contact avec les liquides est du Chlorure de Polyvinyle.

Made in Canada
Fabriqué au Canada

Baxter
Baxter Corporation
Toronto, Ontario,
Canada
88-36-01-003
04/2001

©Copyright
1997, 2001
Baxter Healthcare
Corporation.
All rights reserved.
Tous droits réservés.

0 85412 04160 5

FIGURE 7.1A Intravenous administration equipment Clayton, B.D. (2001). *Basic Pharmacology for Nurses* (12th ed., p. 106). Philadelphia: W.B. Saunders.

FIGURE 7.1B Continu-Flo Solution Set Baxter Corporation, Toronto, Ontario.

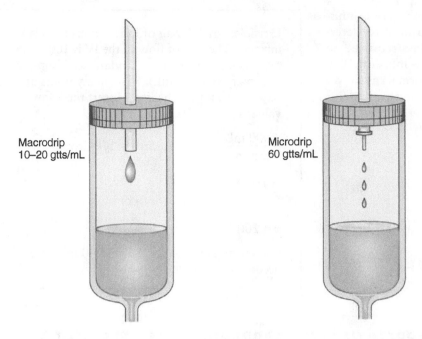

FIGURE 7.2 IV tubing calibration
LeFever Kee, J., & Marshall, S.M. (2000). *Clinical Calculations* (4th ed., p. 185). Philadelphia: W.B. Saunders.

For gravity drips, the rate can be converted to drops per minute using a simple formula.

Formula Statement:

$$\frac{\text{Volume of fluid (mL)}}{\text{Time to infuse (min)}} \times \text{Calibration of IV set (drops/mL)}$$

$$= \text{Rate of flow (drops/min)}$$

Example: Order: Give 1 L over 6 h.

Volume of fluid is 1 L or 1000 mL.

Time to infuse is 6 hours or (6 × 60 min) 360 minutes.

Assume a standard or macrodrip set: 10 drops/mL

Substitute the known values into the formula; be sure to include the units of measurement to ensure an accurate problem statement. Round to the nearest whole number.

$$\frac{1000 \text{ mL (volume)}}{360 \text{ min (time)}} \times 10 \text{ drops/mL (calibration)} = 28 \text{ drops/min (rate)}$$

Sometimes an IV is infusing and you need to determine the time required to complete the infusion. You can use the formula as shown in this following example.

Example: A 1-L bag of intravenous fluid is infusing. The rate of flow of the IV is 100 drops/min, using a macrodrip/standard set (drop factor of 10 drops/mL). How many hours are required to infuse the litre? Insert the known values into the formula and solve.

$$\frac{1000 \text{ mL}}{x \text{ min}} \times 10 \text{ drops/mL} = 100 \text{ drops/min}$$

$$\frac{10\,000}{x} = 100$$

$$x = 100$$

Therefore, 100 min (or 1 h and 40 min) are needed to infuse 1 L.

▶ INTERPRETATION OF ABBREVIATIONS RELATED TO INTRAVENOUS THERAPY

Before proceeding to Exercise 7.1, review the terms related to intravenous therapy in Table 7.1.

TABLE 7.1 Terminology Related to IV Therapy

Term/Abbreviation	Definition/Expansion
bolus	injection of medication over a short period of time
D5W	solution of 5% dextrose in water
D5NS	solution of 5% dextrose in normal saline
NS	solution of normal (0.9%) saline
RL	Ringer's lactate
LVI	large-volume infusion (e.g., 500–1000 mL)
SVI	small-volume infusion (e.g., 25-, 50-, or 100-mL minibag)
minidrip	also called *microdrip*: 60 drops/mL
macrodrip	also called *regular* or *standard drip*: may be 10, 15, or 20 drops/mL; check IV tubing package
IVPB	intravenous piggyback
gtt(s)	drop(s)

▶ EXERCISE 7.1

Complete the following exercise without referring to the above text. State the rate of flow in whole numbers. Correct your answers by using the answer guide starting on page 192. (Value: 1 mark each)

1. Order: 1 L of normal saline over 8 h. Calculate the rate of flow in drops per minute using a regular set with a drop factor of 10 drops/mL.

2. Order: 1000 mL to run at 50 drops per minute. How many hours should this litre infuse using a minidrip (the drop factor is 60)?

Order: 500 mL of 5% dextrose over 4 hours. Answer questions 3 and 4.

3. Calculate the rate of flow in drops per minute using a regular set (the drop factor is 10).

4. Calculate the rate of flow in drops per minute using a minidrip set (the drop factor is 60).

5. The blood transfusion is infusing at 25 drops per minute, and the set is calibrated at 15 drops/mL. What is the hourly infusion rate in millilitres?

6. The I/O record shows that the patient received 3 L over the past 24 h. Calculate the hourly infusion rate.

7. The ordered dose of a drug is dissolved in 100 mL to be infused over 1 h. Calculate the rate of flow in drops per minute using a regular drip set (the drop factor is 10).

8. A 500-mL IV is infusing at the rate of 25 mL/h. How many hours will it take for this IV to be infused?

9. Ampicillin has been added to 50 mL of normal saline. The drug should be infused in 20 min. Calculate the rate of flow in drops per minute using a regular set with a drop factor of 1 mL = 10 drops.

10. A litre of IV fluid has been running at 125 mL/h for 3.5 h. How much remains in the IV container?

11. The IV is ordered to run at 50 mL/h. The administration set delivers 60 drops/mL. Calculate the infusion rate in drops per minute.

12. The IV container is labelled "infuse at 100 mL/h." The administration set delivers 10 drops/mL. The IV is running at a rate of 20 drops per minute. *Is this correct?*

13. An IV container of 500 mL has infused for 1 h at a rate of 100 mL/h. A new rate of infusion is ordered at 50 mL/h. Calculate the number of hours during which the remaining fluid will infuse.

14. The order is for 500 mL of blood over 3 h. Calculate the rate of flow in drops per minute using a set with a drop factor of 15.

15. The IV is infusing at 125 drops/min with a regular set (10 drops/mL). How long will it take to infuse 250 mL?

| Your Score: | /15 | = | % |

▶ CONTINUOUS INTRAVENOUS MEDICATION ADMINISTRATION

Many medications are given by the IV route, which ensures complete absorption of the drug and rapid onset of action. Many institutions use an admixture program in which the drug in the IV solution is prepared and labelled by the pharmacist and administered by the nurse. In other institutions, the nurse must add the drug to the IV solution. Intravenous administration requires a knowledge of medications, mathematics, compatibility, and aseptic technique. Only the main points related to the skills of calculation are addressed in this module.

CRITICAL POINT

It is essential to confirm the compatibility of the medication with the IV solution. Always check the package insert for specific instructions.

To deliver continuous IV medication, follow the instructions for preparing the IV solution and calculate the rate of flow. In some settings, it is policy to use an infusion controller to deliver IV fluids with medications. Always check the policies in the clinical setting. Many adverse reports related to medication administration involve infusion controller devices. Training is required to avoid errors. See Module 9 for information on these electronic devices.

▶ PREPARATION AND CALCULATION OF INTRAVENOUS MEDICATIONS FOR INTERMITTENT ADMINISTRATION

In many situations, a medication is not given continuously. Instead, the drug is added to a small volume of fluid and infused over a short period.

CRITICAL POINT

Intravenous administration is direct and is not retrievable. Too rapid a rate can cause serious adverse effects. Always check the literature carefully or consult the pharmacist before preparing and administering a drug by the IV route.

The medication is added to a secondary intravenous container; this is called a piggyback setup (IVPB) (see Figure 7.3). This setup allows intermittent infusion of the medication over a short duration. The primary solution maintains the IV site or provides additional fluid. Sometimes a reconstitution device is used to add a medication to a minibag (see Figure 7.4). This device provides the advantages of immediate reconstitution without an additional volume of liquid being added to the minibag. It also reduces the risk of contamination during the process of medication preparation.

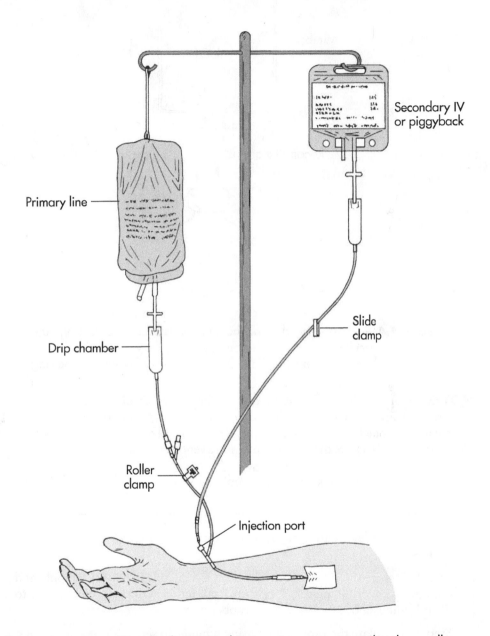

FIGURE 7.3 Intravenous Piggyback (IVPB) administration setup. Note that the smaller container is hung higher than the primary container.
Morris Gray, D.C. (1994). *Calculate with Confidence* (2nd ed., p. 301). Philadelphia: Mosby.

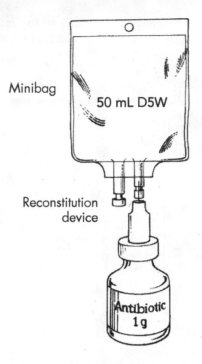

FIGURE 7.4 Reconstitution device. The minibag is squeezed, forcing fluid into the vial. The powder and fluid are mixed thoroughly. Next, the vial and minibag are inverted, and the minibag is squeezed until the fluid from the vial flows into the bag.

NOTE: You are advised to consult a text on the fundamentals of nursing (for example, J. Ross-Kerr and M. Wood, *Canadian Fundamentals of Nursing*, 2nd ed., 2001) or a pharmacology practice text (for example, Richard A. Lehne, *Pharmacology for Nursing Care*, 4th ed., 2001) for the technique of intravenous therapy.

Study the sample problems and then complete Exercise 7.2.

Example: Order: methylprednisolone 80 mg in 50-mL NS infused over 30 min by IVPB

Step 1: Prepare the medication. The drug is available in a 1-mL ampule at a concentration of 80 mg/mL. Draw up 1 mL into a syringe, and inject it into a 50-mL minibag of NS through the rubber port.

Step 2: Calculate the rate of flow using a minidrip set.

$$\frac{\text{Volume (mL)}}{\text{Time (min)}} \times \text{Calibration (gtts/mL)} = \text{Rate of flow (gtts/min)}$$

$$\frac{50}{30} \times 60 = 100$$

The rate is 100 gtts/min.

Example: Order: ampicillin 500 mg in 50 mL D5W infused over 20 min

Step 1: Prepare the medication. The label of a 1-g vial of ampicillin states, "Add 3.5 mL sterile water to yield a solution of 250 mg/mL."

Known ratio: 250 mg/1 mL

Unknown ratio: 500 mg/x mL

$$250:1 = 500:x$$

$$x = (500 \div 250) = 2$$

Draw up 2 mL of drug solution and add it to a 50-mL minibag.

Step 2: Calculate the rate of flow using a regular set.

$$\frac{50 \text{ mL}}{20 \text{ min}} \times 10 \text{ gtts/mL} = 25$$

The rate is 25 gtts/min.

CRITICAL POINT

Intravenous bags are usually overfilled by 5% due to the manufacturing process and to allow some fluid to fill the tubing set. For most clinical situations, this small volume is not significant.

When a medication solution is added to an IV bag, the volume may be increased slightly. Again, in many clinical situations, this is not significant. However, small-volume changes can be very significant for some patients; for example, newborns, very small children, and seriously ill adults. You will learn more about small-volume infusions in Modules 9 and 10.

Now that you have learned how to prepare a medication for IV administration, review the steps in Table 7.2.

TABLE 7.2 Review of Intravenous Administration

Steps	Example of Actions
1. Determine the dose to administer.*	Order is for ampicillin 500 mg in a 50-mL minibag infused over 30 min. As per instructions on the medication label, add 3.5 mL of sterile water to the vial and mix thoroughly to produce a solution of 250 mg/mL.
2. Prepare the IV solution.	Add 2 mL of the drug solution to a 50-mL minibag.†
3. Calculate the rate of flow in drops/min using a regular set (drop factor = 10 gtts/mL). Round the rate of flow to the nearest whole number.	$\dfrac{\text{Volume (mL)}}{\text{Time (min)}} \times \text{Calibration (gtts/mL)}$ $= \text{Rate (gtts/min)}$ $\dfrac{50 \text{ mL}}{30 \text{ min}} \times 10 \text{ gtts/mL}$ $= 17 \text{ gtts/min}$

* Review the reconstitution of powdered drugs as outlined in Module 6.
† Review the calculation of doses for parenteral administration as outlined in Module 6.

▶ **EXERCISE 7.2**

Answer the questions without referring to the above text. Express the rate of flow in whole numbers. Correct your answers by using the answer guide starting on page 192. (Value: 1 mark each)

1. Penicillin 500 000 units is added to 100 mL and the rate of flow is 125 mL/h. Calculate the time in minutes to infuse the drug. The drop factor is 10.

Read the product literature for cefazolin sodium (Ancef) below and answer questions 2 to 5.

Vial Size (mg)	Diluent	Volume to Be Added to Vial (mL)	Approximate Available Volume (mL)	Nominal Concentration (mg/mL)
500	sodium chloride injection or sterile water for injection	2 3.8	2.2 4	225 125
1000	sterile water for injection	2.5	3	334

For intermittent or continuous intravenous infusion. Reconstitute as directed above. SHAKE WELL. Then further dilute reconstituted Ancef in 50 to 100 mL of sterile water for injection or one of the above solutions for intravenous infusion.

2. Describe the reconstitution to yield a solution of 125 mg/mL.

3. If 2 mL of diluent is added to the 500-mg vial, what is the final available volume?

4. Using the concentration of the drug in question 3, calculate the volume to withdraw for a dose of 250 mg. Round to the nearest tenth.

5. The label on the 1000-mg vial states that 2.5 mL of sterile water for injection was added. Calculate the amount to withdraw for a dose of 500 mg. Round to the nearest tenth.

Study the label in Figure 7.5 and answer questions 6 to 10.

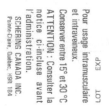 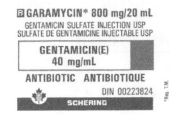

FIGURE 7.5
Schering Canada Inc., Pointe-Claire, Quebec.

6. State the brand name.

7. State the concentration in milligrams per millilitre.

8. What is the total volume?

9. The order is gentamicin sulfate 80 mg IV q8h. A 50-mL minibag with a drop factor of 12 is available. Calculate the amount of drug to add to the minibag.

10. For the order in question 9, calculate the rate of flow in drops per minute to deliver the drug in 20 min.

Your Score:	/10	=	%

CRITICAL POINT

Administration by the intravenous route involves several steps. Review:
- Read the order and the label carefully.
- Prepare the medication by creating a solution (weight-to-volume).
- Calculate the amount to withdraw (usually to the nearest tenth).
- Validate.
- Prepare the IV solution (volume-to-volume solution).
- Calculate the rate of flow (in whole numbers).

▶ **EXERCISE 7.3**

Answer the questions without referring to the above text. Express the rate of flow in whole numbers. Round calculations to the nearest tenth unless otherwise directed. Correct your answers by using the answer guide starting on page 192. (Value: 1 mark each)

Study the labels in Figure 7.6 and answer questions 1 to 15.

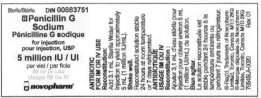
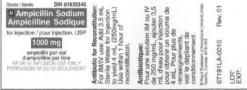

FIGURE 7.6
Novopharm Limited, Toronto, Ontario.

1. Describe the reconstitution of the penicillin.
2. State the resulting concentration of the penicillin.
3. How long is the drug product stable after reconstitution?
4. Calculate the following order, using any method: penicillin G sodium 750 000 IU stat IV. Round to the nearest hundredth.
5. Validate your answer for question 4 by using another method.
6. For the order in question 4, describe the preparation of the intravenous solution, using a 50-mL minibag. State the concentration of this volume-to-volume solution.
7. For the order in question 4, calculate the rate of flow in drops per minute to deliver the drug in 30 min; the drop factor is 10.
8. Describe the reconstitution of the ampicillin.
9. State the resulting concentration of the ampicillin sodium.
10. How long is the drug product stable after reconstitution?
11. Calculate an order of ampicillin 400 mg IV q6h.
12. Validate your answer for question 11 by using another method.
13. For the order in question 11, describe the preparation of the intravenous solution, using a 50-mL minibag. State the concentration produced.
14. For the order in question 11, calculate the rate of flow, in drops per minute, to deliver the drug in 20 min; the drop factor is 12.
15. For the order in question 11, calculate the rate of flow in millilitres per hour.

Your Score:	/15	=	%

▶ EXERCISE 7.4

Answer the questions without referring to the above text. Express the rate of flow in whole numbers. Round calculations to the nearest tenth. Correct your answers by using the answer guide starting on page 192. (Value: 1 mark each)

Study the label in Figure 7.7 and answer questions 1 to 3.

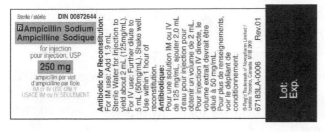

FIGURE 7.7
Novopharm Limited, Toronto, Ontario.

1. Describe the preparation for IV administration.
2. Calculate an order of ampicillin sodium 250 mg IV q6h administered over 20 min.
3. Calculate the rate of flow in drops per minute if the order in question 2 is added to a 25-mL minibag and the drop factor is 10.

Study the labels in Figure 7.8 and answer questions 4 to 15.

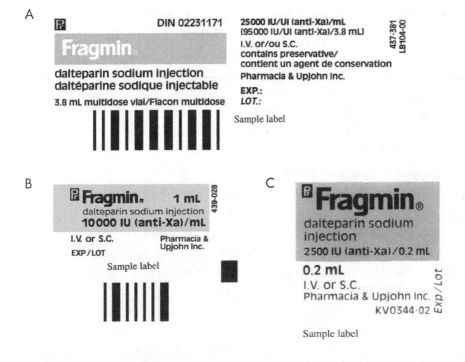

FIGURE 7.8
Pharmacia Canada Inc., Mississauga, Ontario.

4. State the trade name.

5. State the generic name.

Compare the concentration and the volume of the three products, and complete the table.

Label	Concentration	Volume in Vial
A	(6)	(7)
B	(8)	(9)
C	(10)	(11)

12. Using the product in Figure 7.8B, calculate the following order: Fragmin 5000 IU as a loading IV dose.

13. Using the product in Figure 7.8B, calculate the following order: Fragmin 800 IU by continuous IV infusion over 1 h.

14. Using the product in Figure 7.8C, calculate the following order: Fragmin 650 IU as a loading IV dose.

15. Place the products in order from the greatest to the lowest concentration.

Your Score:	/15 =	%

▶ **CASE STUDIES**

Read each clinical situation presented below and answer the questions as indicated. Round the rate of flow to the nearest whole number. Correct your answers by using the answer guide starting on page 192. (Value: 1 mark each)

Mrs. Jones is receiving ampicillin 500 mg IV q4h. An admixture of ampicillin 500 mg in a 50-mL minibag is available. The drop factor is 10 gtts/mL. The drug should infuse over 30 min. The primary IV is running at 125 mL/h.

Calculate the answers to questions 1 to 4.

1. State the rate of flow in drops per minute for the primary IV.

2. State the rate of flow to infuse the drug.

3. What total amount of ampicillin will the patient receive in 24 h?

4. Calculate the total volume of fluid infused in 24 h, including the minibags and the primary IV solution. (Recall that the primary infusion is stopped while the minibag with the medication is running.)

Mrs. A.J. is a 49-year-old patient. She has a primary intravenous infusion of D5W running at 100 mL/h. She is also receiving the following:

cefotetan 1.5 g q12h delivered in a 50-mL minibag of D5W over 30 min at 0600 h and 1800 h

methylprednisolone 80 mg q8h in a 50-mL minibag of NS over 30 min at 0800 h, 1600 h, and 2400 h

Calculate the answers to questions 5 to 8.

5. What is the total amount of NS delivered in 24 h?

6. What is the total amount of D5W delivered in 24 h?

7. How much cefotetan is administered each day?

8. How much methylprednisolone does Mrs. A.J. receive in a 24-h period?

The patient is receiving amikacin 500 mg in 200 mL of NS infused over 1 h.

Calculate the answers to questions 9 and 10.

9. Calculate the rate of flow in drops per minute (the drop factor is 15 gtts/mL).

10. What is the concentration of the drug (in milligrams per millilitre)?

Your Score: /10 = %

▶ POST-TEST

Instructions

1. Write the post-test without referring to any resources.

2. Be careful to

a. Include the appropriate units of measure with the answer when necessary.

b. Round decimal numbers to the nearest whole number for IV rates of flow.

c. Write decimal numbers correctly, using a zero to the left of the decimal point when necessary.

3. Correct the post-test by using the answer guide starting on page 192. (Value: 1 mark each)

1. Calculate the rate of flow in drops per minute for an order of 500 mL over 3 h. The drop factor is 10.

2. Using an administration set with a drop factor of 15 and an infusion rate of 15 gtts/min, how much time would be required to infuse 60 mL?

3. A 100-mL minibag infusion at 50 gtts/min (the drop factor is 60) is initiated at 1130 h. At what time should it be completely infused?

4. An IV is infusing at 125 mL/h. How many millilitres will be absorbed in a 12-h shift?

5. An IV infuses at 20 gtts/min (the drop factor is 10) for 4 h. How much fluid has infused?

Order: cephalothin sodium loading dose of 2 g IV before surgery
Supply: a vial labelled "1 g of cephalothin sodium with 63 mg of sodium per gram." The instructions are to dilute the drug with 2 mL of sterile water for injection and add to the IV solution. The IV of NS is infusing at 100 mL/h.

Answer questions 6 to 8.

6. Describe the reconstitution of the required amount of drug to provide the loading dose.

7. State the rate of flow of the IV if the infusion set delivers 10 gtts/mL.

8. State the amount of sodium the patient will receive from the drug with this loading dose.

Order: amphotericin B (Fungizone) 35 mg IV
Supply: vial with 50 mg and instructions to add 10 mL of sterile water for injection to produce a concentration of 5 mg/mL. Add to 500 mL of D5W and run over 4 h.

Answer questions 9 and 10.

9. Calculate the amount of drug to add to the IV bag.

10. Calculate the rate of flow in drops per minute (the drop factor is 10 gtts/mL). Round to the nearest whole number.

Order: continuous infusion of flumazenil (Anexate) 0.2 mg/h
Supply: 5- and 10-mL ampules of a concentration of 0.1 mg/mL. Add drug to 100-mL minibag and infuse at 20 mL/h.

Answer questions 11 and 12.

11. State the amount of drug to add to the 100-mL minibag to produce a drug concentration of 0.1 mg/mL.

12. Calculate the rate of flow in drops per minute (the drop factor is 60 gtts/mL).

Order: Septra 12 mL IV infused over 90 min
Instructions: dilute each 5 mL of Septra in 75 mL of NS intravenous solution

Answer questions 13 and 14.

13. Calculate the amount of NS intravenous solution required to achieve the recommended dilution.

14. Calculate the rate of flow in drops per minute (the drop factor is 10 gtts/mL).

15. The order is for gentamicin (Garamycin) 375 mg IVPB daily. The drug is available in a vial labelled "80 mg/2 mL." Calculate the rate of flow in drops per minute (drop factor is 60 gtts/mL) to deliver the drug in 30 min.

Order: meperidine (Demerol) 20 mg IV q1h prn
Supply: 25-mg/mL ampule

Answer questions 16 and 17.

16. Calculate the amount to administer.

17. Calculate the amount of drug that is wasted.

18. The order is for furosemide (Lasix) 120 mg IV. The drug is available in a vial labelled "10 mg/mL." The total volume in each vial is 2 mL. Calculate the amount to add to the IV.

19. The order is for pantoprazole 8 mg/h by continuous infusion. The drug is available in a vial containing 40 mg. Add one vial to a 100-mL minibag. Calculate the rate of flow in millilitres per hour.

20. The order is for Kefurox 500 mg IV tid. The drug is available in a 750-mg vial with instructions to add 7.5 mL to yield a solution with a concentration of 100 mg/mL. Calculate the amount to add to the minibag.

21. The order is for Dalacin C 900 mg q8h IV. The drug is available in a vial containing 2 mL and labelled "300 mg." Calculate the amount to add to the minibag.

22. The order is for cefazolin sodium (Ancef) 250 mg IV q8h. The drug is available in a 1-g vial with instructions to add 2.5 mL of diluent to yield a solution with a concentration of 334 mg/mL. Calculate the amount to add to the minibag. Round to the nearest hundredth.

23. The order is for penicillin G sodium 3 million units q6h IV. The drug is available in a vial labelled "5 000 000 units" with instructions to add 3.1 mL of sterile water to yield a total volume of 5 mL. Calculate the amount to add to the minibag.

24. You have prepared a 500-mL bag of NS by adding 5 ampules of Ostac. Each 10-mL ampule contains 30 mg/mL of drug. Calculate the amount of drug added to the IV bag.

25. The order is for an IV of 500 mL over 6 h. It is initiated at 1300 h. At 1500 h, 125 mL have infused. Recalculate the rate of flow in millilitres per hour to complete the infusion on time.

| **Your Score:** | /25 | = | % |

Did you achieve 100%?

YES — Proceed to Module 8.

NO — Analyze your areas of weakness and review this module; then rewrite the post-test. If your score is still less than 100%, please seek remedial assistance.

Drug Dosage Protocols and Special Procedures

▶ MODULE TOPICS

- Mixing of two medications in one syringe
- Sliding scale insulin protocol
- Drug dosage protocols
  - Heparin protocol for stroke
  - Warfarin sliding scale
- Administration by enteral tubing

▶ INTRODUCTION

This module provides an opportunity to learn the skills involved for more complex calculations, including the technique of mixing two medications in the same syringe. A trend in medication administration is the use of protocols to guide calculation and titration of frequently changing doses. A sample protocol for heparin administration provides the example for this skill. This module also provides a clinical simulation of dosage calculations through a case study.

▶ MIXING OF TWO MEDICATIONS IN ONE SYRINGE

In some situations, two medications are drawn into the same syringe for injection. This minimizes discomfort to the patient. You are advised to consult a fundamentals text[1] to review the procedure (e.g., aseptic technique, choosing the correct size of syringe). This section reviews the steps for accurately calculating the dose when two medications are combined in a single syringe.

CRITICAL POINT

Always check compatibility before mixing any medications. When mixing two types of insulin, use a careful technique to avoid contaminating one insulin with the other.

When mixing two medications, you must calculate the dose of each and determine the final volume that must be drawn into the syringe. If the medication is available in a multidose vial, air must be injected into the vial before withdrawal of the medication. The steps of this procedure are outlined in Box 8.1. (**NOTE:** For an explanation of insulin preparations, refer to a current pharmacology text.)[2] Figure 8.1 illustrates the steps for mixing two insulin preparations. Review the steps of the procedure and the example.

---

[1]Ross-Kerr, J., & Wood, M. (2001). *Canadian Fundamentals of Nursing* (2nd ed.). Toronto: Mosby.
[2]Lehne, R.A. (2001). *Pharmacology for Nursing Care* (4th ed.). Toronto: Mosby.

BOX 8.1 Procedure for Mixing Two Types of Insulin

1. Check the medication order for the type and dose of each type of insulin.

2. Check the label on each insulin bottle for the correct drug and the expiry date.

3. Gently roll longer-acting or modified (cloudy) insulin between palms; check that the crystals dissolve and do not adhere to the inside of the bottle. (If the suspension does not mix well, return the bottle to the pharmacy.)

4. Clean the top of each insulin bottle with an alcohol swab. Allow it to dry. **NOTE:** You must clean the rubber diaphragm each time the needle enters it.

5. Draw air into the syringe equal to the dose of the modified (longer-acting, cloudy) insulin (see Step I in Figure 8.1).

6. Insert the needle into the rubber stopper of the modified insulin vial and inject air (see Step II in Figure 8.1). Withdraw the needle.

7. Draw air into the syringe equal to the dose of the short-acting or regular (clear) insulin (see Step III in Figure 8.1).

8. Insert the needle into the rubber stopper of the regular (clear) insulin vial and inject air (see Step IV in Figure 8.1).

9. Withdraw the dose of regular or short-acting (clear) insulin (see Step V in Figure 8.1).

10. Check that the dose is accurate. Expel any air bubbles.

11. Insert the needle into the modified or longer-acting (cloudy) insulin bottle and slowly withdraw the dose (see Step VI in Figure 8.1). **NOTE:** The volume in the syringe should now equal the combined dose of the regular and the modified insulin.

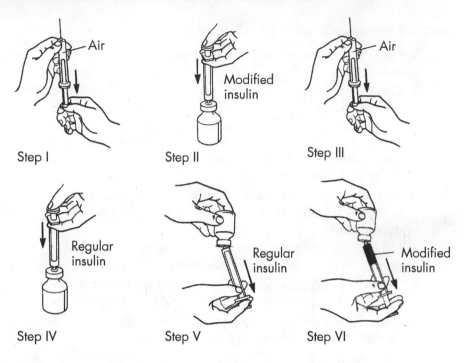

FIGURE 8.1 Mixing of two insulin preparations

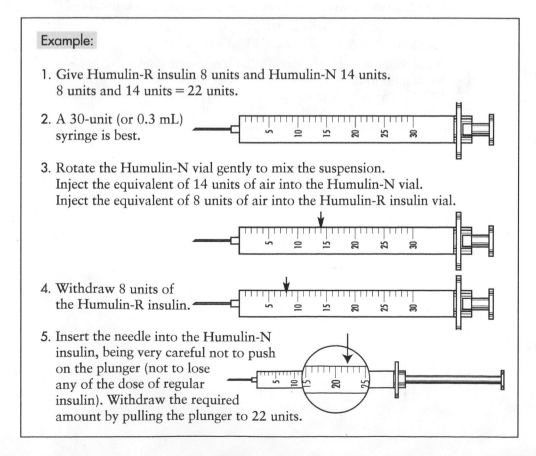

Example:

1. Give Humulin-R insulin 8 units and Humulin-N 14 units.
   8 units and 14 units = 22 units.

2. A 30-unit (or 0.3 mL) syringe is best.

3. Rotate the Humulin-N vial gently to mix the suspension.
   Inject the equivalent of 14 units of air into the Humulin-N vial.
   Inject the equivalent of 8 units of air into the Humulin-R insulin vial.

4. Withdraw 8 units of the Humulin-R insulin.

5. Insert the needle into the Humulin-N insulin, being very careful not to push on the plunger (not to lose any of the dose of regular insulin). Withdraw the required amount by pulling the plunger to 22 units.

You have just learned how to mix two types of insulin in one syringe. Other medications may be drawn up together in one syringe for injection. For example, meperidine (Demerol) may be mixed with dimenhydrinate (Gravol) in a single syringe for IM injection. The steps are outlined in this example.

Example: Order: meperidine (Demerol) 75 mg and dimenhydrinate (Gravol) 50 mg IM

Supply: 2-mL ampule labelled Demerol 50 mg/mL

      1-mL ampule labelled Gravol 50 mg/mL

Calculate the dose for each medication (using ratio/proportion or the formula):

      Volume of Demerol = 1.5 mL

      Volume of Gravol = 1 mL

      Total volume = 2.5 mL

      Select a 3-mL syringe.

Procedure: Draw up 1.5 mL of Demerol from the ampule (discard the remaining 0.5 mL according to agency policy). Draw up 1 mL of Gravol from the 1-mL ampule for a total volume of 2.5 mL.

▶ SLIDING SCALE INSULIN PROTOCOL

Recall that insulin is measured in units and that a unit is the amount of insulin that lowers blood glucose. In the regulation of diabetes mellitus, the patient and the health care professional must find the right amount of insulin to maintain blood glucose within normal limits. The patient may require insulin administration that is based on frequent blood glucose readings. The procedure is often referred to as *sliding scale insulin protocol.*

▶ EXERCISE 8.1

Review the following client situation and then answer the questions below. Correct your answers by using the answer guide starting on page 192. (Value: 1 mark each)

John is newly diagnosed with diabetes mellitus. He is 32 years old, is married, and has one child. He attends a day program to learn to monitor his blood glucose and adjust his insulin dose accordingly. He does a blood glucose test before each meal and at bedtime. In the morning, he takes 10 units of Humulin-N. John's sliding scale protocol is described in Table 8.1.

TABLE 8.1 Sliding Scale Insulin Protocol[‡]

Blood Glucose Level (mmol/L)[§]	Amount of Humulin-R Insulin (units)
< 5	0
5–8	3
8.1–10	4
10.1–12	5
12.1–14	7
14.1–16	8
16.1–18	9
18.1–20	10
> 20	Notify a health care professional

[‡] This sliding scale protocol is provided for teaching purposes only. Always consult recent references before administering any drug.

[§] In countries using SI measurements for lab values, the blood glucose is measured in millimoles per litre (mmol/L). In the United States, the lab value may be expressed as mg/dL. The conversion factor is 0.05551. For example, the normal range is 62–110 mg/dL, which is converted to 3.4–6.1 mmol/L ($62 \times 0.05551 = 3.4$).

CRITICAL POINT

Note that insulin syringes are available in various sizes: 0.3 mL, 0.5 mL, and 1 mL. You should choose the most appropriate size depending on the amount of insulin to be administered.

PART I

Study the labels in Figure 8.2 for morphine and atropine and then answer questions 1 to 3.

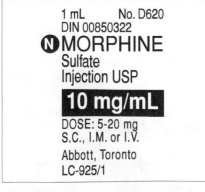

FIGURE 8.2

Morphine sulfate: Reprinted with permission of Abbott Laboratories Limited, Montreal, Quebec. Atropine: Bioniche Pharma Group, London, Ontario

Order: morphine 8 mg IM and atropine sulfate 400 mcg IM 1 h preoperatively

1. Calculate the dose of morphine.
2. Calculate the dose of atropine.
3. Calculate the total volume in the syringe after the 2 drugs are drawn up.
4. In this example, does it matter which drug is drawn up first?

PART II

The table in question 5 shows John's blood glucose readings for two days. Study the table, and refer to the sliding scale protocol to determine the correct insulin dose (Humulin-R).

5. Complete the table by adding the insulin dose.

Time	Blood Glucose (mmol/L)	Insulin Dose (units)
Day One		
ac lunch	15.4	(a)
ac supper	4.7	(b)
hs	12.8	(c)
Day Two		
ac lunch	18.4	(d)
ac supper	8.1	(e)
hs	9.7	(f)

6. Shade the syringe to show the dose given ac lunch on the second day.

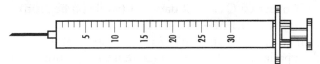

Calculate the total amount of insulin that John received each day.

7. Insulin received on day one.
8. Insulin received on day two.

PART III

Practise the steps of mixing two types of insulin.

9. Order: regular insulin 10 units and NPH 18 units

Procedure: Rotate suspension to ensure homogeneous mixture. Inject equivalent of (a)_____ units of air into NPH vial. Inject equivalent of (b)_____ units of air into regular insulin vial. Withdraw (c)_____ units of (d)_____ insulin and then withdraw (e)_____ units of (f)_____ insulin for a total of (g)_____ units.

10. Order: Humulin-R insulin 8 units and Humulin-N insulin 25 units

Procedure: Rotate suspension to ensure homogeneous mixture. Inject equivalent of 25 units of air into (a)_____ vial; inject equivalent of 8 units of air into (b)_____ vial. Withdraw (c)_____ units of (d)_____ insulin and then withdraw (e)_____ units of (f)_____ insulin for a total of (g)_____ units.

Your Score:	/10	=	%

▶ DRUG DOSAGE PROTOCOLS

With the development of new pharmacotherapies, some medication administration has become more complex. Health care professionals are expected to use evidence-based practice, relying on information from research studies and quality improvement programs. For some drugs, protocols are developed by experts and used in the clinical setting to ensure standards of care. This section of the module introduces you to the experience of calculating dosages according to written protocols: one for the use of heparin for stroke and the other a warfarin sliding scale.

Heparin Protocol for Stroke

The following information illustrates the use of a dosing protocol. Although the most significant information is included, the protocol is not complete and should not be relied on in this format. It is included here for teaching purposes only.[3]

- Patient weight in kg: _____
- Collect APTT,[4] INR,[5] CBC[6] (platelets) before commencing therapy. Then collect APTT every 6 hours until two consecutive APTTs are in goal range — then collect APTT daily. Collect CBC every 2 days × 5 (while on heparin).
- Goal of therapy is APTT 55–69.9 seconds.
- Start heparin infusion 50 units/mL (25 000 units in 500 mL D5W). Commence at rate based on patient weight at 12 units/kg/h to a maximum of 1800 units/h. Use the formula statement or use the dosing chart for stroke protocol (Table 8.2).
- Adjust heparin dosage according to the nomogram in Table 8.3.

---

[3]The Heparin Protocol for Stroke is adapted from the protocol developed by a large regional health authority. Other heparin protocols exist for cardiology and for venous thromboembolism. This information is included to teach the principles of following drug dosing protocols. It should not be used for therapeutic purposes.
[4]activated partial thromboplastin time
[5]international normalized ratio
[6]complete blood count

TABLE 8.2 Heparin Dosing Chart for Stroke Protocol

Weight (kg)	Dosage (mL/h)*
40.1–45	10
45.1–50	11
50.1–55	13
55.1–60	14
60.1–65	15
65.1–70	16
70.1–75	17
75.1–80	19
80.1–85	20
85.1–90	21
90.1–95	22
95.1–100	23
100.1–105	25
105.1–110	26
Continues > 150	—

*The calculated rates are the average for the corresponding weight.

TABLE 8.3 Nomogram for Intravenous Rate of Heparin Administration

APTT (s)	Rate Change
< 35	↑rate by 3 mL/h (150 units/h)
35–44.9	↑rate by 2 mL/h (100 units/h)
45–54.9	↑rate by 1 mL/h (50 units/h)
55–69.9	No change
70–84.9	↓ rate by 1 mL/h (50 units/h)
85–100	Stop infusion for 30 min, then ↓ rate by 2 mL/h (100 units/h)
> 100	Stop infusion for 1 h, then ↓ rate by 4 mL/h (200 units/h)

The following formula statement is used to calculate the rate of flow in millilitres per hour.

Formula Statement:

$$\frac{\text{Weight (kg)} \times 12 \text{ units/kg/h}}{50 \text{ units/mL}} = x \text{ mL/h}$$

NOTE: The IV solution is 50 units/mL, and the maximum rate is 1800 units/h.

Example: Mr. H. is being treated for stroke. His weight is 65.8 kg. You prepare the IV solution according to the instructions. Study the labels in Figure 8.3. Select the 500-mL bag of heparin with 25 000 units. This solution has a concentration of 50 units/mL. Using the formula, you calculate the rate of flow for Mr. H.:

$$\frac{65.8 \text{ kg} \times 12 \text{ units/kg/h}}{50 \text{ units/mL}} = x \text{ mL/h}$$

$x = 16$

Recall: The IV solution is 50 units/mL, and the maximum rate is 1800 units/h.

You initiate the IV at 16 mL/h using an infusion controller device. Mr. H. is receiving 800 units of heparin hourly (16 mL per hour at 50 units/mL). Compare your calculation with the dosing chart in Table 8.2, and note that the rate of flow is the same.

Six hours later, Mr. H.'s lab results are reported. His APTT value is 47.5 s. Using the nomogram in Table 8.3, you find that you must increase the infusion rate by 1 mL/h, and you adjust the infusion controller device to deliver 17 mL/h. Now, Mr. H. is receiving 850 units of heparin hourly, well within the maximum allowed (1800 units/h). However, his APTT value has not reached the desired goal (55–69.9 s). In another six hours, Mr. H.'s APTT value is 56.2 s, and the IV rate is maintained at 17 mL/h. However, six hours later, his APTT is now 71.3 s and the IV rate must be reduced by 1 mL/h (according to the nomogram). The rate is now 16 mL/h, and he is receiving 800 units of heparin hourly.

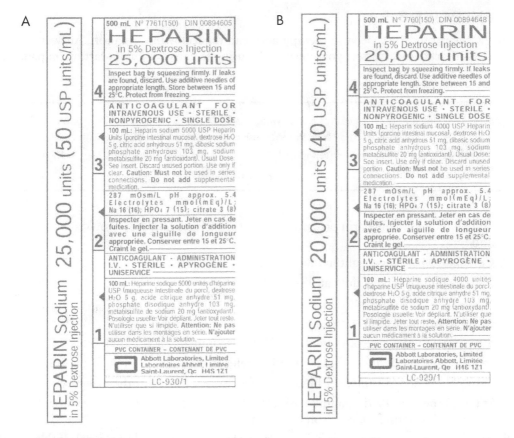

FIGURE 8.3
Reprinted with permission of Abbott Laboratories Limited, Montreal, Quebec.

Warfarin Sliding Scale

Like the heparin protocol, some clinical settings also have protocols for the administration of warfarin, an oral anticoagulant. An example of such a protocol is illustrated in Table 8.4.

TABLE 8.4 Warfarin Sliding Scale

INR Value	Warfarin Dose (mg)
< 1.4	10
1.4–1.99	5
2.00–3.00	2.5
> 3	0

Now test your understanding of using protocols by completing Exercise 8.2.

▶ **EXERCISE 8.2**

Review the protocol for heparin therapy and read the following situation. Answer the questions that follow. Correct your answers by using the answer guide starting on page 192. (Value: 1 mark each)

Mrs. R. is being treated for a stroke. Her weight is 110 pounds. The heparin IV infusion is initiated at 0915 h. At 1315 h, the lab results show the APTT at 40 s. The rate is adjusted accordingly. Six hours later, at 1915 h, the APTT is reported at 52 s, and the rate is adjusted.

---

1. State which of the heparin products illustrated in Figure 8.3 you would choose, and why.
2. Calculate Mrs. R.'s weight in kilograms.
3. State the initial rate of flow at 0915 h:
   a. By using the formula
   b. By using the dosing chart in Table 8.2
4. State the adjusted rate of flow at 1315 h (refer to the nomogram in Table 8.3).
5. State the adjusted rate of flow at 1915 h (refer to the nomogram in Table 8.3).
6. State the number of units per hour that Mrs. R. is receiving at the new rate.
7. State (a) the total IV fluid intake from 0915 h to 1915 h and (b) the total number of units of heparin received from 0915 h to 1915 h.
8. Your patient is receiving warfarin according to the sliding scale protocol. If the INR is 1.42, what dose of warfarin would be given? (Refer to Table 8.4.)
9. Warfarin is available as Warfilone 5-mg scored tabs. Calculate a dose of 7.5 mg.
10. Review the heparin label in Figure 8.3B. The product is running at 23 mL/h. How much heparin is the patient receiving per hour?

Your Score: /10   =   %

▶ **ADMINISTRATION BY ENTERAL TUBING**

Enteral (or tube) feeding is used for patients who are unable to take any nourishment by mouth. For short-term use, the tube may be inserted into the nose (a nasogastric [NG] tube) or mouth (an orogastric tube). For longer-term use, a tube is surgically inserted into the stomach (via gastrostomy) or jejunum (via jejunostomy). Enteral feedings may be given by intermittent or continuous drip. For intermittent or bolus feedings, the amount of solution administered is usually 200 mL or less. Similar to the intravenous method, the enteral feeding can be administered by a gravity drip or an infusion pump. The rate of flow is calculated in drops per minute or in millilitres per hour, depending on the administration device. For continuous administration, a standard schedule for enteral feeding may be set at 50 mL/h and increased as tolerated and as necessary. Enteral feedings may be given at full strength or diluted, depending on the patient's response.

Diluted solutions are referred to as percentages; therefore, you must calculate the amount of water to add to the commercial formula to obtain the desired solution. The following example illustrates the steps.

Example: A patient is to receive a 50% enteral feeding via an NG tube. The order is for 200 mL q4h to run over 30 min. Recall that percent means *portion out of 100*; therefore a 50% solution means 50 parts of feeding formula in 100 parts of solution. Since 50% of 200 mL equals 100 mL, you would add 100 mL of commercial formula to 100 mL of water (for a total volume of 200 mL). You would calculate the rate of flow (in millilitres per hour), attach the tubing to an infusion pump, and set the rate.

Calculation: 200 mL in 30 min

200 mL:30 min $= x$ mL:60 min

$x = 400$ mL/h

Enteral tubes can also be used to administer medications that are in liquid form. The dose is calculated, and the amount is instilled followed by 20 mL of normal saline to flush the tubing and to ensure that the medication reaches the stomach for absorption. See the example below.

Example: Order: morphine 10 mg NG q4h prn

Supply: MOS (morphine oral solution) in a concentration of 10 mg/mL

Give 1 mL of MOS-10 and flush with 20 mL NS.

▶ EXERCISE 8.3

Answer questions 1 to 5. Correct your answers by using the answer guide starting on page 192. (Value: 1 mark each)

1. Order: digoxin 0.1875 mg NG daily
   Supply: elixir labelled "0.05 mg/mL"
   Calculate the amount to administer via an NG tube.
2. Order: furosemide 60 mg NG bid
   Supply: solution in a concentration of 10 mg/mL
   Calculate the amount to administer via an NG tube.
3. Order: morphine 6 mg NG q4h prn
   Supply: MOS in concentrations of 1 mg/mL, 5 mg/mL, and 10 mg/mL
   Calculate the amount to administer; state the concentration used.
4. The order for enteral feeding states, "give 50 mL/h of a 75% solution."
   Calculate how to prepare a sufficient solution for administration over 4 h.

5. Order: omeprazole 20 mg NG bid

   Supply: solution in a concentration of 2 mg/mL

   Calculate the amount to administer via an NG tube.

Your Score:	/5	=	%

CRITICAL POINT

To ensure accuracy, you should calculate the dose using one method and then validate it using another method. You may wish to use a calculator to validate your answer.

▶ EXERCISE 8.4

This exercise provides an opportunity to test your understanding of the concepts presented in this module. Answer the questions without referring to the above text, unless otherwise directed. Correct your answers by using the answer guide starting on page 192. (Value: 1 mark each)

1. You are mixing two medications in one syringe. You have checked a recent pharmacology reference to determine compatibility. One medication is available in an ampule; the other medication is available in a multi-dose vial. Which medication would you withdraw first? Why?

2. You are mixing two insulin preparations in one syringe. One insulin product is clear and short-acting (or rapid-acting), and the other is cloudy and modified (or long-acting). Which insulin product do you withdraw first? Why?

3. You are mixing two medications in one syringe: the volume of the first medication is 0.56 mL, and the volume of the second medication is 0.47 mL. If it is acceptable to round to the nearest tenth, what size syringe will you use?

4. Some individuals with diabetes regulate their insulin administration based on frequent blood glucose readings. This procedure is referred to as _____.

Refer to Table 8.1 (page 126) and answer questions 5 to 7.

5. The patient's blood glucose reading is 11.3 mmol/L. How many units of Humulin-R insulin should be given?

6. The patient's blood glucose reading is 20.1 mmol/L. What action should be taken?

7. The patient's blood glucose reading is 4.9 mmol/L. What action should be taken?

Study the label in Figure 8.4 and answer questions 8 to 10.

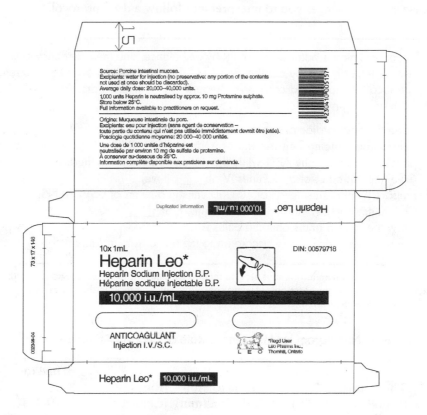

FIGURE 8.4
Leo Pharma Inc., Thornhill, Ontario.

8. The order is for heparin 3500 units sc stat. Calculate the amount to administer.

9. A colleague has withdrawn 0.6 mL from the ampule and asks you to check the dosage. The order states, "heparin 5500 units IV." *Is the dosage correct?*

10. You have withdrawn 0.7 mL of heparin. How many units are contained in this volume?

Your Score: /10 = %

▶ **CASE STUDY**

This case study challenges you to interpret and follow a drug protocol.

A 56-year-old man is admitted to the ER by ambulance, and the emergency physician orders "IV heparin therapy cardiac protocol." The man weighs 68.3 kg. You refer to the protocol* (below) and commence heparin therapy. You administer the bolus at 0800 h and begin the infusion at 0815 h.

Heparin therapy cardiac protocol:
1. Before commencing heparin therapy, draw APTT, INR, Hb (hemoglobin), and platelets. Draw a daily APTT while the patient is on heparin therapy.
2. Give heparin bolus of 5000 units IV at _____ (time).
3. Prepare IV infusion solution of 10 000 units in 500 mL of D5W or NS.
4. Commence heparin infusion at 1000 units/h at _____ (time).
5. Draw the APTT 8 hours after the bolus is administered.
6. Adjust the heparin dosage according to the nomogram in Table 8.5.

---

* This protocol is based on an intravenous heparin therapy cardiac protocol from a regional health authority. It is used here for teaching purposes only. Always consult recent references in the clinical setting before administration of any medication.

TABLE 8.5 Nomogram for Intravenous Rate of Heparin Administration

Therapeutic Ratio	APTT (s)	Length of Time to Stop Infusion (min)	Rate Change	Time to Repeat APTT Test
< 1.5	< 46	0	+10 mL/h +200 units/h	after 8 h
1.5–1.8	46–54.9	0	+5 mL/h +100 units/h	after 8 h
1.9–2.8	55–85.9	0	None	after 8 h
2.9–3.6	86–110	30	−5 mL/h −100 units/h	8 h after restarting heparin
> 3.6	> 110	60	−10 mL/h −200 units/h	8 h after restarting heparin

Answer the questions using the protocol in the case study. Study the label in Figure 8.4. Correct your answers by using the answer guide starting on page 192. (Value: 1 mark each)

1. Using the drug product in Figure 8.4, calculate the volume required to administer the heparin bolus.

2. Calculate the concentration of the IV infusion solution prepared.

3. Calculate the rate of flow in millilitres per hour to deliver the ordered dose of 1000 units/h.

4. At 1615 h, a lab worker calls and reports the APTT at 44 s. State the rate change, and calculate the new rate of flow in millilitres per hour of the IV infusion.

5. At the new rate of flow, how many units of heparin are infused every hour?

6. At 0015 h on the following morning, blood is drawn for APTT. At 0030 h, a lab worker reports the APTT value at 55.8. State the rate change for the infusion.

7. Eight hours later, the APTT is 91. State the rate change, and calculate the new rate of flow in millilitres per hour of the IV infusion.

8. Calculate the total amount of heparin that the patient received from admission to 0815 h on the second day.

9. Calculate the total amount of IV solution the patient received from admission to 0815 h on the second day.

10. Determine how many IV infusions were prepared and infused during the 24-h period.

Your Score:	/10	=	%

▶ POST-TEST

Instructions

1. Write the post-test without referring to any resources.

2. Correct the post-test by using the answer guide starting on page 192. (Value: 1 mark each)

Read the case study below and complete the table.

Mary has had diabetes for several years. She is admitted to the hospital with a severe infection and is placed on the sliding scale insulin protocol. Her insulin orders are as follows:

If blood glucose is 10–15 mmol/L, give 5 units of Humulin-R.
If blood glucose is 15.1–20 mmol/L, give 8 units of Humulin-R.

Time	Blood Glucose Reading (mmol/L)	Insulin Dose
ac breakfast	9.7	(1)
ac lunch	19.3	(2)
stat 1430 h	4.6	(3)
ac supper	15.9	(4)
hs	13.8	(5)

Review the formula for calculating the heparin IV administration rate and answer questions 6 to 10.

$$\frac{\text{Weight (kg)} \times 12 \text{ units/kg/h}}{50 \text{ units/mL}} = x \text{ mL/h}$$

RECALL: The IV solution is 50 units/mL, and the maximum rate is 1800 units/h.

---

6. Calculate the rate of flow for a patient weighing 45.7 kg.
7. Calculate the rate of flow for a patient weighing 189 lbs.
8. What is the maximum rate of flow that can be used according to the heparin protocol?
9. Mr. J. weighs 148 kg. Calculate the rate of flow. Does this exceed the recommended maximum?
10. The IV is set at 17 mL/h. How many units of heparin is the patient receiving each hour?

Order: tinzaparin sodium (Innohep) 175 units/kg sc
Supply: 20 000 units/2 mL
The patient weighs 85 kg. Answer questions 11 and 12.

11. Calculate the dose for this patient.
12. Calculate the amount to give. Round to the nearest hundredth.
13. A patient's lab results have returned and show an elevated INR. An order is given for phytonadione (vitamin K) 1 mg sc stat. It is available in an ampule labelled "10 mg/mL." Calculate the amount to give.
14. The order is for heparin 5000 units sc bid. The available supply is a multidose vial of 5 mL. The concentration is 10 000 units/mL. Calculate the amount to give.

Read the following protocol for the administration of dalteparin sodium (Fragmin) and answer questions 15 to 20. Study the label in Figure 8.5. Do all calculations for a patient weighing 87.3 kg.

Protocol for the administration of dalteparin sodium (Fragmin)

Options for treatment:

1. Administer 200 IU/kg of body weight once a day sc.

2. Administer 100 IU/kg of body weight two times a day sc.

3. Administer a dose of 200 IU/kg of body weight as a continuous intravenous infusion over 24 h.

Instructions for IV infusion: add 10 000 IU to 500 mL of NS or D5W in a glass or plastic container. The solution should be used within 24 h.

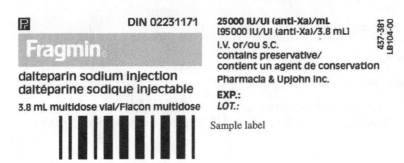

FIGURE 8.5

Pharmacia Canada Inc., Mississauga, Ontario

15. For option 1 in the protocol, calculate the dose.

16. For option 1 in the protocol, calculate the volume to administer. Round to the nearest hundredth.

17. For option 2 in the protocol, calculate the volume to administer for a single dose. Round to the nearest hundredth.

18. State the concentration of the IV infusion in international units per millilitre.

19. Calculate the IV dose in international units per hour. Round to the nearest whole number.

20. Calculate the rate of flow in millilitres per hour to deliver the IV dose. Round to the nearest whole number.

Order: meperidine 60 mg and hydroxyzine 30 mg IM

Supply: meperidine in ampules of 10 mg/mL, 25 mg/mL, 50 mg/mL, 75 mg/mL, and 100 mg/mL; Atarax (hydroxyzine) 50 mg/mL

Answer questions 21 to 23.

21. Calculate the volume of meperidine. State the concentration you are using.

22. Calculate the volume of hydroxyzine.

23. State the total volume in the syringe.

24. Order: Humulin-R 13 units and Humulin-N 25 units sc stat. The available supply is both types of insulin in a concentration of 100 units/mL. Calculate the total volume to administer.

25. The order is 15 units Humulin 30/70 sc stat. Refer to the label in Figure 8.6. Calculate the volume to administer.

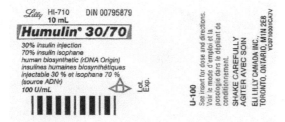

FIGURE 8.6

Your Score: /25 = %

Did you achieve 100%?

YES — Proceed to Module 9.

NO — Analyze your areas of weakness and review this module; then rewrite the post-test. If your score is still less than 100%, please seek remedial assistance.

Calculations of Dosages for Pediatric and Geriatric Patients

► **INTRODUCTION**

In every clinical situation involving medication administration, accurate dosage calculation is an important responsibility. Neonatal, pediatric, elderly, and acutely ill patients require very precise dosage administration. This module does not present any new mathematic principles, but it does provide information specific to dosage calculations for children and older adults.

► **HOW TO DECREASE ERRORS IN DOSE FOR INFANTS AND CHILDREN**

"Tenfold overdoses in premature infants are a well-documented error."[1] Reading this statement causes us to pause and consider the potentially serious outcomes of human error. In one study, a substantial number of trainees made tenfold errors in calculations for infants and small children.[2] You must take all precautions to calculate, validate, and then examine the answer with the attitude that you are looking for errors. For example, read the following order from a patient record: "Dose 100 microgram/kg, weight 800 g, prescribed dose 800 micrograms."[3] The correct dose is 80 mcg. *What went wrong?* The health care professional forgot to convert grams to kilograms. Perhaps you spotted the error immediately by assuming that human error must be anticipated. Experts in the field of medication errors advise that we should use a technique developed for the aerospace industry.[4] It is known as *failure mode and effects analysis,* and it involves identifying mistakes that will happen — before they happen. As you read this

---

[1] Caldwell, N. (2000). How to decrease errors in dose. *Journal of Pediatrics, 137*(1), 142.
[2] Rowe, C., Koren, T., & Koren, G. (1998). Errors by paediatric residents in calculating drug doses. *Archives of Disease in Childhood, 79*(1), 56–58.
[3] Ibid.
[4] Cohen, M., Senders, J., & Davis, N. (1994). Failure mode and effects analysis: A novel approach to avoiding dangerous medication errors and accidents. *Hospital Pharmacy, 29*(4), 319–30.

module and complete the exercises, keep in mind that calculations for infants and children often involve converting one measure to another: micrograms to milligrams or milligrams to grams. You can prevent the type of disastrous overdose that might have occurred with the above example.

▶ CALCULATION OF DOSAGES FOR CHILDREN

For adults, standard dose ranges exist, but for children, because of the many factors of age, body weight, and disease factors, the dose is often stated as the amount to give per kilogram of body weight. This requires additional steps of calculation.

CRITICAL POINT

It is your responsibility to calculate and validate the dose calculation and also to confirm that the dose is within the recommended range. Errors in dose can be very serious for infants and children. Develop the habit of always writing down your calculation and asking a colleague to validate it.

Calculations Based on Body Weight

Frequently, a dose for a child is written as an amount of drug per kilogram of body weight, for example, 1 mg/kg q6h. The dose may also be stated as an amount to give in 24 h in a specific number of divided doses. The following example illustrates the steps of calculations based on body weight and the procedure for confirmation, calculation, and validation of the dose for children.

1. Determine the recommended dose from a reliable literature source (i.e., text, package insert, or pharmacy literature).
2. Compare the recommended and the prescribed doses to ensure the prescribed dose is within the recommended range.
3. Calculate the dose for the infant or child.
4. Calculate the amount to administer.
5. Validate your answer.

Example: Order: penicillin G 200 000 units/kg/d q6h

Recommended dose: "dose for children, penicillin G 200 000 units per kg per day in equally divided doses q4–6h"

Compare:	The prescribed dose is within the recommended range.
Recipient:	9-year-old child weighing 32 kg
Calculate the dose:	200 000 units $\times$ 32 kg = 6 400 000 units/d
	q6h = 4 doses
	6 400 000 units $\div$ 4 = 1 600 000 units per dose
	(or 1.6 million units)

Calculate the amount to administer: vial label states "5 million units (5 m units).

Add 3.1 mL diluent to yield a volume of 5 mL."

$$5 \text{ m units:} 5 \text{ mL} = 1.6 \text{ m units:} x \text{ mL}$$

$$5x = 8$$

$$x = (8 \div 5) = 1.6$$

Give 1.6 mL.

Validation: $\dfrac{5 \text{ m units}}{5 \text{ mL}} = \dfrac{1.6 \text{ m units}}{1.6 \text{ mL}}$

$$8 = 8$$

In some situations, the order may state the specific dose to be given for each administration. The steps are similar to the previous example. Let's do another example.

Example: Order: cefuroxime 860 mg IV q8h

Recommended dose: "cefuroxime 50–100 mg/kg/d divided q6–8h"

Recipient:	12-year-old child weighing 34.5 kg
Calculate the dose:	860 mg $\times$ 3 doses = 2580 mg/d
Compare:	dose per kg is 2580 mg/34.5 kg = 74.78 mg/kg (rounded to 75 mg/kg)

The dose of 75 mg/kg is within the recommended range of 50–100 mg/kg.

CRITICAL POINT

This author encourages you to read everything with attention: the order, the label, and the calculation that you write. This cannot be overemphasized. To illustrate how easy it is to overlook things, an exercise is included here. Read the following statement and count the Fs. Then check the answer at the bottom of the page.[5]

FEATURE FILMS ARE THE RESULT OF YEARS OF SCIENTIFIC STUDY COMBINED WITH THE EXPERIENCE OF YEARS.

Medications for children are often prepared in liquid form. Therefore, calibrated measuring devices are commonly used; these include small plastic cups (30 mL or 1 fl. oz.), droppers, measuring spoons, and oral syringes. See Figure 9.1 for illustrations of these devices.

mL = millilitre
oz = ounce
dr = dram
T = tablespoon
tsp = teaspoon

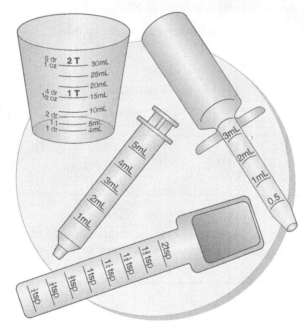

FIGURE 9.1 Calibrated measuring devices
Kee, J., & Marshall, S. (2000). *Clinical Calculations* (4th ed., p. 216). Philadelphia: W.B. Saunders.

▶ PEDIATRIC CASE STUDY

Complete this case study to practise reading package insert literature. Correct your answers by using the answer guide starting on page 192 . (Value: 1 mark each)

---

[5] Answer: you should find six Fs. If not, read the sentence again out loud, or ask someone else to read it and find the Fs.

Jack weighs 32 lb. and is to receive Ancef, 25 mg/kg/d in 3 equal doses.

Use Tables 9.1 and 9.2, the package inserts of Ancef (cefazolin sodium), to answer the questions.

TABLE 9.1 Pediatric Dosage Guide: 25 mg/kg/d

Weight		25 mg/kg/d Divided into 3 Doses		25 mg/kg/d Divided into 4 Doses	
lb.	*kg*	*Approximate Single Dose (mg/q8h)*	*Volume Needed of 125 mg/mL* Solution*	*Approximate Single Dose (mg/q6h)*	*Volume Needed of 125 mg/mL* Solution*
10	4.5	40 mg	0.35 mL	30 mg	0.25 mL
20	9.0	75 mg	0.6 mL	55 mg	0.45 mL
30	13.6	115 mg	0.9 mL	85 mg	0.7 mL
40	18.1	150 mg	1.2 mL	115 mg	0.9 mL
50	22.7	190 mg	1.5 mL	140 mg	1.1 mL

* 125 mg/mL concentration may be obtained by reconstituting the 500-mg vial with 3.8 mL of diluent.

TABLE 9.2 Pediatric Dosage Guide: 50 mg/kg/d

Weight		50 mg/kg/d Divided into 3 Doses		50 mg/kg/d Divided into 4 Doses	
lb.	*kg*	*Approximate Single Dose (mg/q8h)*	*Volume Needed of 225 mg/mL* Solution*	*Approximate Single Dose (mg/q6h)*	*Volume Needed of 225 mg/mL* Solution*
10	4.5	75 mg	0.35 mL	55 mg	0.25 mL
20	9.0	150 mg	0.7 mL	110 mg	0.5 mL
30	13.6	225 mg	1.0 mL	170 mg	0.75 mL
40	18.1	300 mg	1.35 mL	225 mg	1.0 mL
50	22.7	375 mg	1.7 mL	285 mg	1.25 mL

* 225 mg/mL solution may be obtained by reconstituting the 500-mg vial with 2 mL of diluent.

1. What is the frequency of administration for this order?
2. What is the approximate single dose in mg?
3. What volume is needed to deliver this dose?
4. How is the powder reconstituted to produce a concentration of 125 mg/mL?

Calculate questions 5 to 7 without referring to the package inserts, and compare your responses with the previous answers.

5. Based on body weight, what total daily dose would Jack receive?

6. How much should Jack receive for each dose of Ancef?

7. Compare your answers for questions 2 and 6; explain the difference.

8. Refer again to the package inserts. What volume should Jack receive if the frequency is changed to qid?

Your Score:	/8	=	%

▶ EXERCISE 9.1

Complete the following exercise without referring to the above text. Correct your answers by using the answer guide starting on page 192. (Value: 1 mark each)

The recommended dose for a child under 10 years of age is 4 mg/kg/d in 4 equally divided doses, not to exceed 200 mg/d. The recommended dose for a child over 10 years of age is 5 mg/kg/d in 4 equally divided doses, not to exceed 400 mg/d. Answer questions 1 to 4.

1. Noah is 9 years old and weighs 20 kg. Calculate the total recommended daily dose.

2. Calculate each of Noah's doses. Round to the nearest tenth.

3. Francesca is 14 years old and weighs 51.2 kg. Calculate her recommended daily dose. Confirm whether her dose is within the recommended range.

4. Joey is 4 years old and weighs 34.3 lb. Calculate each of his doses. Round to the nearest tenth.

5. Solu-Medrol 8.5 mg IV q6h is ordered for a child who weighs 17 kg. The recommended dose is 0.5–1 mg/kg/dose given q6h. Is the dose within the recommendations?

6. Solu-Medrol is available in an ampule labelled "20 mg/mL." Calculate the volume required to give the dose stated in question 5. Round to the nearest hundredth.

7. The order is for albuterol inhalation 0.15 mg/kg. Makenna weighs 9.1 kg. Calculate the required volume if the drug form available is 5 mg/mL. Round to the nearest hundredth.

The recommended dose for epinephrine is 0.01 mL of a 1:1000-mL solution per kg as a single dose. Available is an epinephrine 1:1000 solution (or 1 mg/mL). Answer questions 8 to 10.

8. Sierra weighs 15 kg and is ordered 10 mcg/kg epinephrine sc stat. Is this within the recommended range?

9. Using the available supply of epinephrine, calculate the amount to administer to Sierra.

10. Shade in the dose on the syringe.

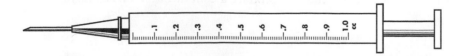

Your Score:	/10	=	%

▶ ADMINISTRATION BY SMALL-VOLUME INFUSION

For intravenous administration to the pediatric client, very small volumes of fluids are infused. See Figure 9.2 for an illustration of the volume control chamber. These chambers are part of the intravenous administration set, and they hold up to 150 mL of fluid. They are useful in administration to infants, children, and adults who cannot tolerate the infusion of large volumes. Note that one set delivers a microdrip (usually 60 drops/mL), and the other set delivers a macrodrip (10, 15, or 20 drops/mL). A desired amount of fluid can be added to the volume control chamber from the IV bag, and then medication can be added to the chamber.

To enhance the accuracy of the rate of administration, electronic delivery devices are used. Figure 9.3 illustrates a volumetric infusion controller and a volumetric infusion pump. An infusion controller works by gravity. The device works by the clamping and releasing of the IV tubing. An infusion pump uses pressure to deliver the desired number of drops per minute (or millilitres per hour). The risk with this latter type of equipment is obvious: infiltration can occur because the pump acts against resistance. Both delivery devices sound warning alarms if any problems occur. Frequent monitoring is essential. Because of the variety of machines available, check the instructions and any procedures in the clinical setting.

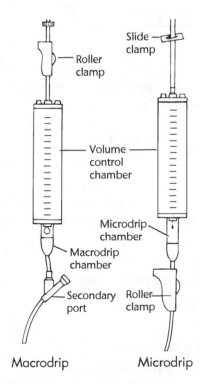

FIGURE 9.2 Intravenous administration sets
Clayton, B.D. (2001). *Basic Pharmacology for Nurses* (12th ed., p. 106). Philadelphia: W.B. Saunders.

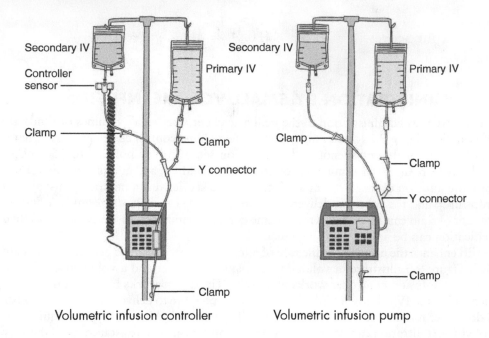

FIGURE 9.3 Intravenous administration sets
LeFever Kee, J., & Marshall, S. (2000). *Clinical Calculations* (4th ed., p. 194). Philadelphia: W.B. Saunders.

CRITICAL POINT

Always check the calibration of an electronic infusion controller; volumetric devices are set in millilitres per hour, and nonvolumetric devices are set in drops per minute.

Read the example and then proceed to Exercise 9.2.

Example: A child weighing 28 kg must be given hydrocortisone by IV infusion. The dose is 1 mg/kg, and the package insert instructions read, "100 mg to 3000 mg may be diluted in 50 mL and infused over 10 minutes." The available supply is Solu-Cortef Act-O-Vial labelled "100 mg/2 mL."

Calculate the dose: $1 \text{ mg/kg} = 1 \times 28 = 28 \text{ mg}$

Calculate the amount: strength of supply is 50 mg/mL

$$50 \text{ mg:1 mL} = 28 \text{ mg:}x \text{ mL}$$

$$50x = 28$$

$$x = (28 \div 50) = 0.56$$

Add 0.56 mL to 50 mL in the small-volume chamber.

Calculate the rate of flow using a set that delivers 10 gtts/mL: answer = 50 gtts/min.

▶ EXERCISE 9.2

The following exercise presents calculations that require administration by small-volume infusion. Complete the exercise without referring to the above text. Remember to calculate and then validate. Correct your answers by using the answer guide starting on page 192. (Value: 1 mark each)

The recommended dose of ampicillin for children under 40 kg is 25–50 mg/kg/d in equally divided doses at 6- to 8-hour intervals. Answer questions 1 to 4 for a child weighing 15 kg.

1. Calculate the safe daily dosage range.

2. Calculate each dose if given q8h.

3. The drug is available in vials of 125 mg, 250 mg, 500 mg, 1 g, and 2 g. For a dose of 250 mg, describe the procedure to reconstitute it and to add it to 20 mL in a small-volume infusion.

4. Calculate the rate to infuse over 20 minutes using a set that delivers 60 gtts/mL.

The recommended loading dose of digoxin for infants 1 month to 2 years is 30–50 mcg/kg divided into three or more doses. The initial dose should be one half of the total. Answer questions 5 to 8.

5. For a 1-year-old infant whose weight is 8.2 kg, calculate the range for the total loading dose.

6. The ampule is labelled "250 mcg/mL." Using the lowest loading dose, calculate the amount to give for the initial dose. Round to the nearest hundredth.

7. Using the highest loading dose, calculate the amount required for the initial dose. Round to the nearest hundredth.

8. For this infant, a loading dose of 40 mcg/kg is ordered and one half of the total dose is administered. Four hours later, you must give one quarter of the loading dose. Calculate the amount.

Order: Run IV at a rate to deliver 1 mg/kg/h. The child weighs 12.5 kg. Answer questions 9 and 10.

9. Calculate the dose required.

10. If the amount is added to 20 mL, calculate the rate of flow in millilitres per hour.

Your Score:	/10	=	%

▶ ADMINISTRATION OF MEDICATIONS IN GERIATRICS

This section briefly reviews the precautions regarding crushing medications, and it presents clinical situations for calculations of medications for older adults. Because of advanced age and the possibility of concomitant physical health problems, older adults are at higher risk for adverse reactions to medications. Due to changes in pharmacokinetics, the aging individual may not excrete medications at the same rate as a younger individual; consequently, the dosages of many medications must be adjusted for older persons. In addition, individuals in their seventh, eighth, and ninth decades of life may have neurological or functional problems that cause difficulty with swallowing. In this instance, oral dosage forms (tablets) may have to be crushed and mixed with a small amount of liquid or soft food such as pudding or applesauce. This book does not undertake to teach the procedures related to drug administration; you should consult a reliable source for more information on the techniques of crushing tablets, mixing medication with liquid or food, and administering medication by an NG tube, if necessary. You must also check sources of information to determine whether milk, water, or juice is best, and whether a drug must be given with food or on an empty stomach.

CRITICAL POINT

Crushing a medication may change its bioavailability and/or its rate of absorption. This can increase the risk of toxicity if the drug dosage is delivered too rapidly (i.e., crushing a product that is designed for slow release). Always consult a pharmacist, the product information, or a reliable reference source before crushing any oral dosage form. Ask whether the drug is available in liquid formulation; this is the most accurate and desirable alternative.

Table 9.3 briefly summarizes types of oral dosage forms and whether they can be crushed.

TABLE 9.3 Oral Medications and Crushing*

Dosage Form	Details Regarding Crushing
tablets	Most uncoated, sugar-coated, or film-coated tablets can be crushed.
capsules — may contain powder, liquid, pellets, or beads. Some are designed for slow release (see the next page). The name of the product may be a warning that it may be slow-release capsules; e.g., *spansules*, *gradumets*, and *timespans*.	Some capsules can be opened and their contents mixed with liquid or food, unless they are designed for slow release. The liquid in the capsule can be withdrawn with an 18-gauge needle. The entire capsule can be dissolved in water (this takes time) and administered.
chewable	These can be crushed.
sublingual or buccal pills	These should not be crushed. They are designed to be absorbed through the blood vessels of the mouth and tongue.

(continued)

*Adapted from Miller, D. (2000). To crush or not to crush. Available on-line through Nursing Library http://www.findarticles.com/cf_0/m3231/mag.jhtml=NursingLibrary

TABLE 9.3 Oral Medications and Crushing* *(continued)*

enteric-coated pills	Do not crush. The coating is designed to prevent absorption in the stomach. Absorption should occur in the intestine.
slow-release or long-acting pills Examples: SR (slow or sustained release) LA (long acting) CR (controlled release) CRT (controlled-release tablet) SA (sustained action) TD (time delay) TR (time release) XL (extended length) Contin (continuous acting)	Do not crush. They are designed for slow absorption over an extended time. Crushing may increase the rate of absorption and cause toxicity or other adverse effects.

▶ **EXERCISE 9.3**

The following exercise presents calculations that occur frequently in settings that provide care to older adults. Complete the exercise without referring to the above text. Remember to calculate and then validate. Correct your answers by using the answer guide starting on page 192. (Value: 1 mark each)

1. Order: triazolam 0.375 mg PO

    Supply: Halcion (triazolam) 0.25-mg scored tablets

    Calculate the number of tablets to give.

Order: pericyazine 15 mg every morning PO and 40 mg every evening PO
Supply: Neuleptil oral solution; each millilitre contains 10 mg of pericyazine
Answer questions 2 and 3.

2. Calculate the volume for the morning dose.

3. Calculate the volume for the evening dose.

4. Order: vitamin D_2 12 000 IU/d

    Supply: Drisdol oral solution; each millilitre contains 8288 IU vitamin D_2

    Calculate the volume to administer. Round to the nearest tenth.

5. Order: Chloral Hydrate 750 mg qhs

    Supply: syrup labelled "500 mg/5 mL"

    Calculate the volume to give.

6. Order: Halcion 0.125 mg PO

    Supply: Halcion 0.25-mg scored tablets

    Calculate the number of tablets to give.

7. Order: prednisone 40 mg PO

   Supply: two dosage strengths: 5-mg scored tabs and 50-mg scored tabs

   Calculate two options to deliver the dose.

The order is for amoxicillin 250 mg q8h. The patient has difficulty swallowing, and the medication is supplied as an oral suspension with the following information on the label: "each 5 mL of strawberry-flavoured suspension contains amoxicillin trihydrate equivalent to 125 mg of amoxicillin." Among the nonmedicinal ingredients is listed sodium 5.95 mg/5 mL. Answer questions 8 and 9.

8. Calculate the amount of suspension to administer for one dose.

9. Calculate the amount of sodium delivered with each dose.

10. Order: haloperidol 500 mcg PO bid

    Supply: haloperidol syrup 2 mg/mL

    Calculate the volume required for the dose. Round to the nearest hundredth.

Your Score:	/10	=	%

Dosage Calculation by Renal Function

Older individuals may have reduced renal function, which can significantly affect drug elimination. Because of this, dosages of some drugs are based on an estimation of renal function. Two examples are provided.

Example: An antiviral drug is administered to residents in long-term care (LTC) centres to prevent influenza type A virus infection. Table 9.4 presents the dosage schedule recommended by the manufacturer. Mrs. Franklin is residing in an LTC centre. Her creatinine clearance is 45. According to the schedule, she would receive 100 mg of the agent every other day.

TABLE 9.4 Dosing Schedule for Antiviral Agent*

Creatinine Clearance (mL/min/1.73 m^2)	Dosing Schedule
> 80 mL/min	100 mg once daily
60–79	alternating daily doses of 100 mg and 50 mg
40–59	100 mg every other day
30–39	100 mg twice weekly
20–29	50 mg three times a week
10–19	alternating weekly doses of 100 mg and 50 mg

* This dosing schedule is provided for teaching purposes only. Always consult drug package information for dosage recommendations.

Example: See Table 9.5 for the dosing schedule for fluconazole (Diflucan). The oral suspension is prepared by mixing the powder with 24 mL of water to produce a concentration of 10 mg/mL. If Mrs. Franklin were prescribed this drug, she should receive 50% of the usual adult dose. For treatment of oropharyngeal candidiasis, the dose is 100 mg/d.

Calculate the dose: 10 mg:1 mL = 50 mg:x mL

$$10x = 50$$

$$x = (50 \div 10) = 5$$

Mrs. Franklin should receive 5 mL to deliver a dose of 50 mg (50% of the usual adult dose).

TABLE 9.5 Dosing Schedule for Fluconazole (Diflucan)

Creatinine Clearance (mL/min/1.73 m²)	Percentage of Usual Adult Dose
> 50	100
21–50	50
11–20	25

▶ EXERCISE 9.4

Complete the exercise without referring to the above text unless otherwise directed. Correct your answers by using the answer guide starting on page 192. (Value: 1 mark each)

Study the labels for Voltaren in Figure 9.4 and answer questions 1 to 4.

1. Which of the products can be crushed?
2. Which of the products could be used for an order of diclofenac sodium 75 mg PO in 3 divided doses? Calculate the amount to give for each dose.
3. What is the maximum daily dose for this medication?
4. Describe the recommended dosage schedule for the treatment of rheumatoid arthritis. Which of the drug products could be used for this schedule?
5. Refer to Table 9.5. The available supply of fluconazole is a 50-mg/mL oral suspension. The usual adult dose is 50 mg. Calculate the dose for Mr. J.P. if his creatinine clearance is 19 mL/min/1.73 m², and the amount to be administered.

Usual adult dosage: *Osteoarthritis:* Initial and maintenance dose is 25 mg three times daily. *Rheumatoid arthritis:* Initially: 25-50 mg three times daily depending on the severity of the condition. For maintenance: 25 mg three times daily or the minimum amount to provide continuous control of symptoms. Maximum daily dose is 150 mg. Tablets should be swallowed whole, with food. Not recommended for use in patients under 16 years of age. Product monograph supplied on request. Protect from heat and humidity. **PHARMACIST: Dispense with the PATIENT INFORMATION LEAFLET provided to you.**

Novartis Pharmaceuticals Canada Inc.
Novartis Pharma Canada inc.
Dorval (Québec) H9S 1A9

℞ **Voltaren® 25mg**
diclofenac sodium tablets
comprimés de diclofénac sodique

DIN 00514004   2551

Ⓥ **NOVARTIS**

Anti-inflammatory analgesic agent
Agent anti-inflammatoire – analgésique

100 enteric-coated tablets
100 comprimés entéro-solubles

Posologie habituelle pour adulte : *Ostéoarthrite:* Dose d'attaque et d'entretien habituelle : 25 mg trois fois par jour. *Arthrite rhumatoïde :* Dose d'attaque : 25 à 50 mg trois fois par jour selon la gravité du cas. Dose d'entretien : 25 mg trois fois par jour ou administrer la dose minimale qui produit un contrôle continu des symptômes. La dose maximale quotidienne est de 150 mg. Les comprimés doivent être avalés entiers, avec de la nourriture. Non recommandé chez les patients de moins de 16 ans. Monographie fournie sur demande. Protéger de la chaleur et de l'humidité. **PHARMACIEN: Remettre avec le feuillet INFORMATION POUR LE PATIENT qu'on vous a fourni.**

Usual adult dosage: *Osteoarthritis:* Initial and maintenance dose is 25 mg three times daily. *Rheumatoid arthritis:* Initially: 25-50 mg three times daily depending on the severity of the condition. For maintenance: 25 mg three times daily or the minimum amount to provide continuous control of symptoms. Maximum daily dose is 150 mg. Tablets should be swallowed whole, with food. Not recommended for use in patients under 16 years of age. Product monograph supplied on request. Protect from heat and humidity. **PHARMACIST: Dispense with the PATIENT INFORMATION LEAFLET provided to you.**

℞ **Voltaren® 50mg**
diclofenac sodium tablets

Anti-inflammatory analgesic agent
Agent anti-inflammatoire – analgésique

Ⓥ **NOVARTIS**

100 enteric-coated tablets
100 comprimés entéro-solubles

DIN 00514012   2561

Posologie habituelle pour adulte : *Ostéoarthrite:* Dose d'attaque et d'entretien habituelle : 25 mg trois fois par jour. *Arthrite rhumatoïde :* Dose d'attaque : 25 à 50 mg trois fois par jour selon la gravité du cas. Dose d'entretien : 25 mg trois fois par jour ou administrer la dose minimale qui produit un contrôle continu des symptômes. La dose maximale quotidienne est de 150 mg. Les comprimés doivent être avalés entiers, avec de la nourriture.

Non recommandé chez les patients de moins de 16 ans. Monographie fournie sur demande. Protéger de la chaleur et de l'humidité. **PHARMACIEN: Distribuer avec le feuillet INFORMATION POUR LE PATIENT qu'on vous a fourni.**

Novartis Pharmaceuticals Canada Inc.
Novartis Pharma Canada inc.
Dorval (Québec) H9R 4P5
3021-11-97A

Adult dose for rheumatoid arthritis and osteoarthritis: Once a maintenance dosage of 75 mg per day has been established with Voltaren® enteric coated tablets, a once-daily dose of Voltaren® SR 75 mg may be substituted, taken morning or evening. Patients on a maintenance dose of 150 mg per day may be changed to a twice daily dose of one Voltaren® SR 75 mg tablet taken morning and evening. Tablets should be swallowed whole with liquid, preferably at mealtime. Maximum daily dose for Voltaren® in any dosage form is 150 mg. Not recommended for use in patients under 16 years of age. Product monograph supplied on request. Store at room temperature and protect from humidity. **PHARMACIST: Dispense with the PATIENT INFORMATION LEAFLET provided to you.**

℞ **Voltaren® SR 75mg**
diclofenac sodium
diclofénac sodique

Anti-inflammatory analgesic agent
Agent anti-inflammatoire – analgésique

Ⓥ **NOVARTIS**

100 slow release tablets
100 comprimés à libération lente

DIN 00782459   2540

Posologie pour adulte dans l'arthrite rhumatoïde et l'ostéo-arthrite: Lorsque la dose d'entretien a été établie à 75 mg par jour avec les comprimés entéro-solubles de Voltaren®, on peut substituer le comprimé Voltaren® SR 75 mg administré une fois par jour, le matin ou le soir. Chez les patients qui prennent une dose d'entretien de 150 mg par jour, on peut la remplacer par une dose biquotidienne de Voltaren® SR 75 mg, soit un comprimé pris le matin et un le soir. Avaler les comprimés entiers avec du liquide, de préférence au repas. La dose maximale de Voltaren® sous

toutes ses formes est de 150 mg par jour. Non recommandé chez les patients de moins de 16 ans. Monographie fournie sur demande. Garder à la température ambiante et à l'abri de l'humidité. **PHARMACIEN: Distribuer avec le feuillet INFORMATION POUR LE PATIENT qu'on vous a fourni.**

Novartis Pharmaceuticals Canada Inc.
Novartis Pharma Canada inc.
Dorval (Québec) H9R 4P5
3019-11-98B

FIGURE 9.4
Novartis Pharmaceuticals Canada Inc., Dorval, Quebec.

Study Figure 9.5 and answer questions 6 to 10.

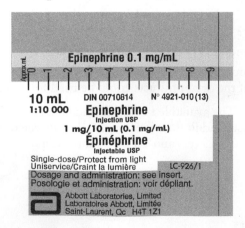

FIGURE 9.5
Reprinted with permission of Abbott Laboratories Limited, Montreal, Quebec.

6. What is the concentration of the drug?

7. What is the total volume contained in the vial?

8. Calculate the volume for a dose of 200 mcg.

9. What is the total amount of drug contained in the vial?

10. Calculate the volume for a dose of 0.25 mg to be administered IV slowly.

| Your Score: | /10 | = | % |

► EXERCISE 9.5

This exercise provides additional practice in calculating dosages for pediatric patients. Complete the exercise without referring to the above text unless otherwise directed. Correct your answers by using the answer guide starting on page 192. (Value: 1 mark each)

1. A supply of erythromycin is a suspension labelled "125 mg/5 mL." Calculate the volume to give for a dose of 80 mg PO. Round to the nearest tenth.

Study the labels in Figure 9.6 and answer questions 2 to 5.

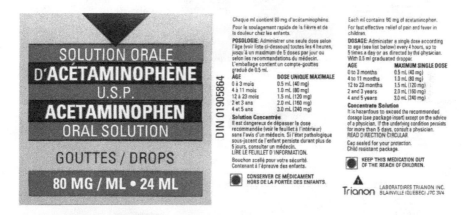

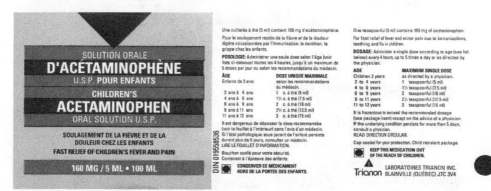

FIGURE 9.6 Two strengths of acetaminophen solution
Trianon Laboratories Inc., Blainville, Quebec.

2. State which solution you are using. Calculate the volume for Patricia, whose weight is 17 kg, if the order is for acetaminophen 10 mg/kg. Round to the nearest tenth.

3. State which solution you are using. Calculate a dose for Colleen, who weighs 37 lb., if the order states, "acetaminophen 15 mg/kg for temperature." Round to the nearest tenth.

4. Read the dosage recommendations on each label. Compare the recommendations for a child aged 4 years.

5. During a home visit, you are asked the following question by Mrs. Johnson. She has purchased the product labelled "80 mg/mL" and has read that she should give 1.5 mL to her child aged 15 months. She asks whether she can use a teaspoon to measure this amount. What is your response?

Study the labels in Figure 9.7 and answer questions 6 to 10.

A

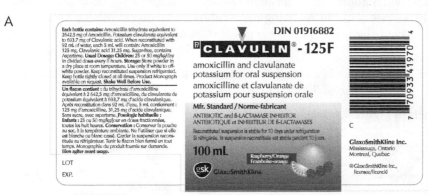

B

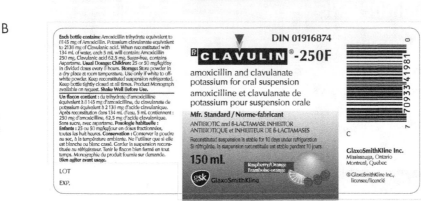

FIGURE 9.7
GlaxoSmithKline, Inc., Mississauga, Ontario.

6. What is the trade or brand name of this drug product?

7. Name the two drug components contained in this product.

8. For the product in Figure 9.7A, what is the strength of amoxicillin in milligrams per millilitre of the solution?

9. For the product in Figure 9.7B, what is the strength of amoxicillin in milligrams per millilitre of the solution?

10. The package insert states that the pediatric dose is based on the amoxicillin component: "give 13.3 mg/kg q12h." Calculate the amount to give per dose to a child weighing 37.1 kg. Round to the nearest whole number.

| Your Score: | /10 | = | % |

▶ GERIATRIC CASE STUDY

Read the case study below and answer the questions, referring to the text where indicated. Correct your answers by using the answer guide starting on page 192. (Value: 1 mark each)

Mrs. K.D. is an 86-year-old woman recently admitted to a long-term care centre. On admission, the medication orders include the following:

clomipramine hydrochloride 10 mg PO daily
commence therapy with baclofen 5 mg PO tid; increase to 10 mg tid after 3 days
"Pink Lady" PO q6h prn

Two weeks after admission, Mrs. K.D. attends a family wedding and is exposed to influenza A virus. She is treated with an antiviral agent. Her lab tests indicate that her creatinine clearance is 57 mL/min/1.73 m^2.

Study the label in Figure 9.8 and answer questions 1 and 2.

Adult dosage: Depression and Obsessive Compulsive Disorder (OCD): Initially 25 mg daily, increase gradually by 25 mg up to 150-200 mg. Severely depressed patients, up to 300 mg daily. Severe cases of OCD, up to 250 mg daily. **Children and adolescents: For OCD treatment only:** Initially 25 mg daily, increase gradually up to a maximum of 200 mg daily. Maintain at lowest effective dose. Product monograph supplied on request. Protect from heat (store between 2 and 30°C).

®**Anafranil**® **10**mg
clomipramine hydrochloride tablets

Antidepressant, Antiobsessional
Antidépresseur, Anti-obsessionnel

Ü NOVARTIS

100 tablets
100 comprimés

DIN 00330566   1116

0 63601 01116 5

Posologie pour adultes: dépression et troubles obsessionnels compulsifs (TOC): Au début, 25 mg par jour; augmenter graduellement par paliers de 25 mg jusqu'à 150 à 200 mg. Dépression sévère, jusqu'à 300 mg par jour. Troubles obsessionnels compulsifs sévères, jusqu'à 250 mg par jour. **Enfants et adolescents en traitement de TOC seulement:** Au début, 25 mg par

jour; augmenter graduellement jusqu'à un maximum de 200 mg par jour. Maintenir à la plus faible dose efficace. Monographie de produit fournie sur demande. Protéger de la chaleur (conserver entre 2 et 30°C).

Novartis Pharmaceuticals Canada Inc.
Novartis Pharma Canada inc.
Dorval (Québec) H9R 4P5
3052-11-97A

FIGURE 9.8
Novartis Pharmaceuticals Canada Inc., Dorval, Quebec.

1. State the trade or brand name of the drug.
2. Calculate the number of tablets for a single dose.

Study the label in Figure 9.9 and answer questions 3 to 5.

3349-11-00A

Usual adult dosage: Titration begins with 5 mg 3 times a day for 3 days, followed by increases to 10, 15, and 20 mg 3 times a day at 3-day intervals. Maximum dose should not exceed 80 mg daily (20 mg 4 times a day). Not recommended in children. If benefits are not evident after a trial period, the medication *should be withdrawn slowly.* Product monograph supplied on request. Protect from heat and humidity.

Novartis Pharmaceuticals Canada Inc.
Novartis Pharma Canada inc.
Dorval (Québec) H9S 1A9

℞**Lioresal®10mg**
baclofen tablets USP
comprimés de baclofène USP

DIN 00455881   1635

Ⓤ **NOVARTIS**

Muscle relaxant, antispastic
Relaxant musculaire, antispastique

100 tablets
100 comprimés

Posologie habituelle pour adulte: Instituer le traitement avec 5 mg 3 fois par jour pour 3 jours; augmenter la dose à 10, 15, et 20 mg 3 fois par jour à 3 jours d'intervalle. La dose maximale ne devrait pas dépasser 80 mg par jour (20 mg 4 fois par jour). L'emploi chez l'enfant n'est pas conseillé. Si après une période d'essai la réponse n'est pas satisfaisante, *le sevrage devrait se faire lentement.* Monographie fournie sur demande. Protéger de la chaleur et de l'humidité.

FIGURE 9.9
Novartis Pharmaceuticals Canada Inc., Dorval, Quebec.

3. State the trade or brand name of the drug.

4. Calculate the number of tablets for a single dose on day 1.

5. State the total amount of baclofen received on the first day of therapy.

6. The instructions for a Pink Lady are as follows: mix Maalox Regular Suspension with lidocaine viscous 2% solution. The proportions are 2:1 (Maalox:Xylocaine). Describe the preparation for a dose of 45 mL PO.

7. Refer to Table 9.4 (page 152) and determine the dosage for the antiviral agent.

Complete the table for administration of baclofen over a period of 4 days. Refer to the label in Figure 9.9.

Baclofen	Days 1 to 3	Day 4
single dose	(8)	(8)
number of tabs/dose	(9)	(9)
total daily dosage	(10)	(10)

Your Score:	/10	=	%

▶ POST-TEST

Instructions

1. Write the post-test without referring to any resources.

2. Be careful to include units with all answers (e.g., milligrams, millilitres, or tablets).

3. Round oral doses to the nearest tenth.

4. Round parenteral doses to the nearest hundredth.

5. Correct the post-test by using the answer guide starting on page 192. (Value: 1 mark each)

1. A child weighing 16.4 kg is to receive 30 mg/kg/d of amoxicillin oral suspension. The available supply is 125 mg/5 mL. The daily dose is to be divided and given q8h. Calculate a single dose.

2. A child is to receive a dose of erythromycin 80 mg PO. Medication containing 125 mg/5 mL is available. Calculate a single dose.

3. The order states, "0.015 mg/kg loading dose of digoxin IV." Calculate the volume required for a child weighing 3.2 kg if the available strength is 0.25 mg/mL.

4. The order for a 10-year-old boy who weighs 34 kg is for atropine sulfate 0.01 mg/kg IM. The literature states that 0.4 mg is the maximum dose that may be given to a child. *Is this order safe?*

5. The order is for phenobarbital 2 mg/kg PO bid. The available strength is 15 mg/5 mL. Calculate the dose in millilitres for a child weighing 19 lb.

6. Order: Lasix 2 mg/kg IV

   Supply: 10 mg/mL

   The infant's weight is 3.9 kg. Calculate the volume to administer.

7. The infant's order is gentamicin 2 mg IV q12h. Gentamicin 20 mg/2 mL is available. Calculate a single dose in millilitres.

Order: ampicillin 50 mg/kg/d SC in 6 divided doses

Supply: ampicillin 125 mg/mL in a 2-mL vial

The infant weighs 11.2 kg. Answer questions 8 to 10.

8. Calculate the total daily dose in milligrams.

9. Calculate a single dose in milligrams.

10. Calculate the amount to give to deliver a single dose.

11. The infant's weight is 860 g, and the order is for morphine 0.6 mg/kg/d SC q4h. The supply available is 2 mg/mL. Calculate the amount to give to deliver a single dose.

12. Shefali is a 9-month-old baby who weighs 7.2 kg. She has received acetaminophen 60 mg PO q4h × 24 h. The literature states that a child under 1 year should receive 15–60 mg/dose q4–6h, not to exceed 65 mg/kg/d. *Has she received more than the daily limit?*

13. Order: captopril 6.25 mg PO

    Supply: quadrisect tablet of 25 mg

    Calculate the number of tablets to give.

14. The order is for lactulose 15 mL tid. The label of a 500-mL bottle reads, "each mL of solution contains 667 mg." How much does the patient receive in each dose?

The patient is to receive a 1-week treatment with dexamethasone (Decadron). The oral dosage form is available in 2 strengths: 0.5-mg scored tablets and 4-mg scored tablets. The solution for injection is 4 mg/mL. Complete the table.

Day	Dose	Amount to Give (include dosage form and strength)
1	4 mg IM	(15)
2, 3	2 mg PO	(16)
4, 5	1 mg PO	(17)
6, 7	0.5 mg PO	(18)

19. Calculate the total amount of dexamethasone received over the course of treatment.

Another patient is to receive dexamethasone but cannot swallow the tablets. The drug is available as an oral syrup that has a concentration of 1 mg/mL. Answer questions 20 and 21.

20. Calculate the amount to administer for the dose on day 2.
21. Calculate the amount to administer for the dose on day 5.
22. Order: vitamin B_{12} 30 mcg daily IM

    Supply: 0.1 mg/mL

    Calculate the amount to inject.
23. The order is for theophylline 300 mg PO q8h. Because the patient cannot swallow pills, an elixir is provided that has a concentration of 80 mg/15 mL. Calculate the amount to administer for a single dose.
24. For the order in question 23, Theo-SR (theophylline) is also available. If the elixir is not available, could you crush this tablet and administer it with water?
25. Order: zopiclone 3.75 mg PO

    Supply: scored tablet of 7.5 mg

    Calculate the number of tablets to give.

Your Score:	/25	=	%

Did you achieve 100%?

YES — Proceed to Module 10.

NO — Analyze your areas of weakness and review this module; then rewrite the post-test. If your score is still less than 100%, please seek remedial assistance.

Calculations for Critical Care

▶ MODULE TOPICS

- Calculation of fluid needs
- Titration of intravenous medications
- Use of calculation tables

▶ INTRODUCTION

Modern technology and methods have increased drug safety through such techniques as electronic infusion pumps, premixed intravenous medication, and unit-dose delivery systems. However, human error still plays a role in mistakes in dosage calculations, and some of these mistakes can be very serious. This module offers additional challenges that occur in settings such as the emergency departments, trauma units, coronary care units, and other settings that provide critical care. The principles remain the same; the calculations may involve additional steps. You may want to complete this unit as a personal challenge or in connection with a relevant clinical placement.

▶ CALCULATION OF FLUID NEEDS

Orders for fluids may be expressed as total volume per day, as millilitres per hour, or according to body weight or surface area. For example, a common recommendation for children is 1500 mL/m^2/d. An alternative guideline is the following:

- 100 mL/kg for the first 10 kg
- 50 mL/kg for the next 10 kg
- 20 mL/kg for all remaining kg

The following examples illustrate these concepts.

Example: Calculate the hourly fluid replacement for a child with a body surface area of 0.6 m^2.

1500 mL/m^2 = 1500 × 0.6

= 900 mL

This child should receive 900 mL/d (or approximately 38 mL/h

[$\frac{900}{24} = 37.5$]).

Example: Calculate the 24-h fluid needs for an individual weighing 60 kg.

For the first 10 kg:
100 mL/kg = 1000 mL

For the next 10 kg:
50 mL/kg = 500 mL

For the remaining kg:
60 − 20 = 40 kg × 20 mL/kg = 800 mL

This individual should receive 2300 mL in 24 h (or approximately 96 mL/h

[$\frac{2300}{24} = 95.8$]).

▶ TITRATION OF INTRAVENOUS MEDICATIONS

Dosages in critical care and emergency units are usually calculated by titration; that is, the dose is adjusted to the patient's condition. The dose is ordered as a weight or volume of drug per kilogram of body weight per unit of time, for example, 5 mcg/kg/min.

Drugs used in these settings are potent, and the flow rate must be carefully and accurately monitored. The drugs are delivered by intravenous piggyback (IVPB), a volutrol or buretrol chamber in the infusion line, and direct IV push. Direct push is the administration of medications into an access port near the venipuncture site. It also refers to administration in less than 10 min. Because of the risks with IV push (or bolus), many clinical settings consider this an advanced competency. Always check agency policy. You must know the right "timing" for IV push; for example, insulin can be given over 1 to 2 min, but adenosine (Adenocard) must be given over 1 to 3 s.

The following two exercises present opportunities to practise titrating medications. The first involves adults in critical care or emergency settings; the second focuses on neonates in critical care. These calculations require a careful, step-by-step approach. You should write out the problem and the solution, then validate your answer. In many instances, nurses are expected to write the calculations directly on the patient's record and validate their answers with a colleague. To calculate the rate of flow of IV medications, you can solve step-by-step using ratio and proportion, or you can use the formula.

Formula Statement:

To determine flow rate for mcg/kg/min (expressed in mL/h):

$$\frac{\text{Amount required (mcg)} \times \text{Weight (kg)} \times 60 \text{ min/h}}{\text{Concentration (mcg/mL)}} = \text{Flow rate (mL/h)}$$

Example: Give dopamine 5 mcg/kg/min.

The patient weighs 61 kg.

Mix 200 mg in 250 mL: concentration = $200 \div 250 = 0.8$ mg = 800 mcg/mL

$$\frac{5 \text{ mcg} \times 61 \text{ kg} \times 60 \text{ min}}{800 \text{ mcg/mL}} = 22.875 \text{ mL/h}$$

The flow rate is 23 mL/h = 23 drops/min (minidrip).

NOTE: The above formula can also be used to calculate an order for milligrams per kilogram per hour. Simply substitute milligrams for micrograms.

Let's do another example. Some settings have flow charts or other helpful tools to assist with these calculations. Examples of these tools are also included in this module. Let's use the tool that follows to calculate a dopamine drip.

Formula Statement for Mixing Dopamine Solution for Infants:

To make 50 mL of solution that provides 5 mcg/kg/min at a rate of 1 mL/h:

5 mcg × ____ kg × 60 min × 50 mL = ____ mcg dopamine in 50 mL of
IV solution

____ mcg ÷ 40 000 mcg/mL = ____ mL dopamine

Dopamine Drip

Using the solution concentration determined above, adjust the IV rate in millilitres per hour as follows:

IV Rate	Dopamine Dosage
0.5 mL/h	2.5 mcg/kg/min
1 mL/h	5 mcg/kg/min
1.5 mL/h	7.5 mcg/kg/min

Example: Order: dopamine 5 mcg/kg/min in D5W at 1 mL/h

The infant weighs 860 g or 0.86 kg

To make 50 mL of solution that provides 5 mcg/kg/min at a rate of 1 mL/h:

5 mcg × 0.86 kg × 60 min × 50 mL

= 12 900 mcg dopamine in 50 mL of IV solution

Supply: dopamine 200 mg/5 mL

40 mg/mL = 40 000 mcg/mL

Calculate the dose of dopamine:

12 900 mcg ÷ 40 000 mcg/mL = 0.32 mL dopamine

Prepare the IV solution and run at 1 mL/h to provide 5 mcg/kg/min.

▶ USE OF CALCULATION TABLES

To assist clinicians with complex calculations, some settings use dosage tables. Read Box 10.1 and the following examples, and then complete Exercise 10.1.

BOX 10.1 Dopamine Dosage

Add 200 mg to 500 mL solution. The concentration is 400 mcg/mL solution.

Find the body weight across the top.

Find the desired dose on the left side.

Follow the line across the table to determine the flow rate in mL/h.

Dose (mcg/min)	Body Weight (kg)									
	50	55	60	65	70	75	80	85	90	95
1	7	8	9	10	11	11	12	13	13	14
2	15	17	18	19	21	23	24	25	27	29
3	23	23	27	29	31	34	36	38	41	43
4	30	33	36	39	42	45	48	51	54	57
5	37	41	45	49	53	56	60	64	67	71

Example: Patient's weight: 65 kg   Find 65 on the top line.

Order: 2 mcg/min   Find 2 on the left side.

The rate is 19 mL/h.

Patient's weight: 69 kg   The closest number on the top line is 70 kg.

Order: 4 mcg/min   Find 4 on the left side.

The rate is 42 mL/h.

Patient's weight: 75 kg   Find 75 on the top line.

Order: 3.5 mcg/min   Find the rates for 3 and 4: the rate for 3 is 34 mL/h, and the rate for 4 is 45 mL/h.

The midpoint is 39.5.

The rate is approximately 40 mL/h.

These above examples can be validated with the formula statement given on page 162.

$$\frac{\text{Amount required (mcg)} \times \text{Weight (kg)} \times 60 \text{ min/h}}{\text{Concentration (mcg/mL)}} = \text{Flow rate (mL/h)}$$

$$\frac{2 \times 65 \times 60}{400} = 19.5 \approx 20 \text{ mL/h}$$

$$\frac{4 \times 69 \times 60}{400} = 41.4 \approx 41 \text{ mL/h}$$

$$\frac{3.5 \times 75 \times 60}{400} = 39.4 \approx 39 \text{ mL/h}$$

Two additional examples are given below to illustrate the use of dosage charts. The first describes the use of an antidote called acetylcysteine (Mucomyst) and the second example illustrates the use of Digibind. A patient is admitted with an overdose of acetaminophen, and treatment is commenced with acetylcysteine (Mucomyst). The drug is available in 10-mL vials and 30-mL vials labelled "20% solution." Recall that a 1% solution refers to 1 g of medication in 100 mL of solution. Therefore, the 20% solution would have 20 g in 100 mL. This converts to 20 000 mg/100 mL, or 200 mg/mL. Table 10.1 summarizes the information found in the medication package insert.

TABLE 10.1 Dosage Chart for Mucomyst*

Body Weight (kg)	Initial Infusion in D5W over 15 min Mucomyst® (mL)	Initial Infusion 5% Dextrose (mL)	2nd Infusion in 500 mL D5W over 4 h Mucomyst (mL)	3rd Infusion in 1 L D5W over 16 h Mucomyst (mL)
10–15	11.25	40	3.75	7.5
15–20	15	50	5	10
20–25	18.75	75	6.25	12.5
25–30	22.5	75	7.5	15
30–40	30	100	10	20
40–50	37.5	200	12.5	25
50–60	45	200	15	30
60–70	52	200	17.5	35
70–80	60	200	20	40
80–90	67.5	200	22.5	45
90–100	75	200	25	50
100–110	82.5	200	27.5	55

* Always refer to the package information. This table is provided for teaching purposes only.

Note that the table has overlapping measurements. For example, if a patient weighs exactly 50 kg, you could choose two lines. For the patient weighing 50.4 kg, use the lesser amount, but for the patient weighing 50.7 kg, use the greater amount.

The following example uses Table 10.1 as a reference.

Let's review the initial infusion for a patient weighing 65 kg. First, you would draw up 52 mL of Mucomyst. You would need to use two 30-mL vials. The Mucomyst would be added to 200 mL of D5W and the solution infused over 15 min. The rate of flow would depend on the drop factor of the administration set.

To perform the second infusion for the same patient, you would draw up 17.5 mL of Mucomyst. You would need one 30-mL vial for this amount. The Mucomyst would be added to 500 mL of D5W and the solution infused over 4 h. Again, the rate of flow would depend on the drop factor of the administration set.

The procedure for the third infusion involves drawing up 35 mL of Mucomyst. You would need one 30-mL vial and half of the 10-mL vial. The Mucomyst would be added to 1000 mL of D5W and the solution infused over 16 h.

Now let's demonstrate how this dosage could be calculated if the dosage table were not available.

Example: Order: Mucomyst 100 mg/kg in 1 L D5W over 16 h

Recall that the vial contains a 20% solution that has a concentration of 200 mg/mL.

The patient weighs 75 kg.

Required dose: 100 mg:1 kg $= x$ mg:75 kg

$$x = 100 \times 75 = 7500$$

The dose is 7500 mg.

Calculate the amount of drug to add to the IV fluid:

$$200 \text{ mg:1 mL} = 7500 \text{ mg:}x \text{ mL}$$

$$200x = 7500$$

$$x = (7500 \div 200) = 37.5 \text{ mL}$$

You would add 37.5 mL to a 1-L bag of D5W and infuse over 16 h. The rate of flow would be $1000 \div 16 = 62.5$ mL/h.

Compare your calculation with Table 10.1. You will note that the chart indicates that 40 mL would be used; this is an average dose for patients between 70 and 80 kg. Although it is more accurate to do the calculation, the doses in the table are within a safe range.

What would you do if you wanted to know how much drug the patient is receiving every hour? The IV solution contains 7500 mg in 1000 mL or 7.5 mg/mL. To calculate the amount of drug received every hour, multiply the rate of flow by the concentration: $62.5 \times 7.5 = 468.75$ mg. You might also calculate it in the following way. The litre contains 7500 mg of drug and will be infused in 16 h. The per-hour rate of drug delivery would be the total amount of drug divided by the time for delivery: $7500 \div 16 = 468.75$ mg.

In the emergency department you may treat individuals who have overdosed on drugs. The following example involves a digoxin overdose, which is treated with Digibind. Each vial of the drug will bind approximately 0.5 mg of digoxin.

Example: A patient ingested 25 tablets of digoxin, and each tab contains 0.25 mg. It is estimated that 80% of the drug is absorbed. How many vials of Digibind would be required?

Amount of drug ingested: 25 tabs $\times$ 0.25 mg = 6.25 mg

Amount of drug absorbed: 6.25 mg $\times$ 80% (or 0.8) = 5 mg

Number of vials required: 1 vial binds 0.5 mg = x vials bind 5 mg

$$0.5x = 5$$

$$x = 10$$

Ten vials are required for treatment.

To check that you understand these calculations, answer the questions in Exercise 10.1.

▶ EXERCISE 10.1

Complete the following exercise. Correct your answers by using the answer guide starting on page 192. (Value: 1 mark each)

Refer to Table 10.1 (page 165) for questions 1 to 7.

A patient weighing 22 kg is receiving the initial infusion with 18.75 mL of Mucomyst. Answer questions 1 and 2.

1. How many milligrams will this patient receive in this first infusion?
2. How many millilitres of D5W will be infused?

A patient weighing 52 kg has the initial infusion running. Answer questions 3 to 5.

3. What is the total volume in the IV bag?
4. Over what time should this IV infuse?
5. What is the rate of flow in drops per minute if the IV set delivers 10 gtts/mL? Round to the nearest whole number.
6. For a patient weighing 78 kg, the third infusion has been running for 6 h. How many grams of drug have been delivered in that time (assuming the IV is on time)?
7. Calculate the concentration of the initial infusion for a patient weighing 10 kg (what is the drug concentration in milligrams per millilitre of D5W)?

Questions 8 to 10 refer to the use of Digibind. For each of the situations in questions 8 to 10, assume that 80% of the drug is absorbed. Round to the nearest whole number. Each vial of Digibind will bind approximately 0.5 mg of digoxin.

8. The patient ingested 38 tablets of 0.25-mg strength. How many vials of Digibind would be required?

9. The patient ingested 30 tablets of 125-mcg strength. How many vials of Digibind would be required?

10. The patient ingested 50 tablets of 0.0625-mg strength. How many vials of Digibind would be required?

Your Score:	/10	=	%

CRITICAL POINT

Complex calculations sometimes involve interpreting complex labels. For example, the drug concentration can be expressed in many ways. The medication label may indicate the strength or concentration of a drug available in solution. The strength may be stated as a percentage or a ratio. For example, a 1% solution is 1 g of medication in 100 mL of solution.

Review the following example. Study the label in Figure 10.1. The label provides the following information:

- Drug name: lidocaine hydrochloride
- Total volume in the container: 250 mL
- Total amount of drug in the container: 2 g
- Drug concentration expressed in milligrams per millilitres and as a percent: 8 mg/mL or 0.8%
- Intravenous solution: dextrose injection USP
- Usual adult dose: "Administer at a rate of 1–4 mg lidocaine HCl/min. Do not exceed 300 mg/hour."

Read the label carefully. What else can you learn about the product and precautions?

CRITICAL POINT

When solving complex calculations, always approach the problem by using the same steps:

1. Know the dose required. If necessary, convert units (e.g., milligrams to micrograms).
2. Know the drug concentration. If necessary, convert units.
3. Calculate the rate of flow in drops per minute or millilitres per hour. Round your answer to the nearest whole number.
4. Validate your answer by "working backward." Accept a reasonable rounding error.

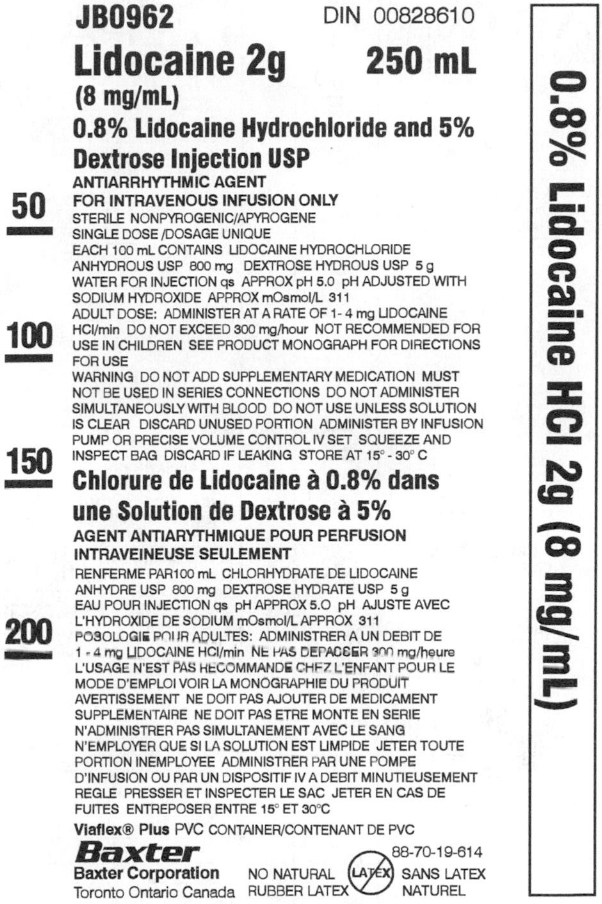

JB0962 DIN 00828610

Lidocaine 2g   250 mL
(8 mg/mL)

0.8% Lidocaine Hydrochloride and 5% Dextrose Injection USP

ANTIARRHYTHMIC AGENT

50

FOR INTRAVENOUS INFUSION ONLY
STERILE NONPYROGENIC/APYROGENE
SINGLE DOSE /DOSAGE UNIQUE
EACH 100 mL CONTAINS LIDOCAINE HYDROCHLORIDE
ANHYDROUS USP 800 mg DEXTROSE HYDROUS USP 5 g
WATER FOR INJECTION qs APPROX pH 5.0 pH ADJUSTED WITH
SODIUM HYDROXIDE APPROX mOsmol/L 311
ADULT DOSE: ADMINISTER AT A RATE OF 1- 4 mg LIDOCAINE

100

HCl/min DO NOT EXCEED 300 mg/hour NOT RECOMMENDED FOR
USE IN CHILDREN SEE PRODUCT MONOGRAPH FOR DIRECTIONS
FOR USE
WARNING DO NOT ADD SUPPLEMENTARY MEDICATION MUST
NOT BE USED IN SERIES CONNECTIONS DO NOT ADMINISTER
SIMULTANEOUSLY WITH BLOOD DO NOT USE UNLESS SOLUTION
IS CLEAR DISCARD UNUSED PORTION ADMINISTER BY INFUSION
PUMP OR PRECISE VOLUME CONTROL IV SET SQUEEZE AND
INSPECT BAG DISCARD IF LEAKING STORE AT 15° - 30° C

150

Chlorure de Lidocaine à 0.8% dans une Solution de Dextrose à 5%

AGENT ANTIARYTHMIQUE POUR PERFUSION INTRAVEINEUSE SEULEMENT

RENFERME PAR100 mL CHLORHYDRATE DE LIDOCAINE
ANHYDRE USP 800 mg DEXTROSE HYDRATE USP 5 g
EAU POUR INJECTION qs pH APPROX 5.0 pH AJUSTE AVEC
L'HYDROXIDE DE SODIUM mOsmol/L APPROX 311

200

POSOLOGIE POUR ADULTES: ADMINISTRER A UN DEBIT DE
1 - 4 mg LIDOCAINE HCl/min NE PAS DEPASSER 300 mg/heure
L'USAGE N'EST PAS RECOMMANDE CHEZ L'ENFANT POUR LE
MODE D'EMPLOI VOIR LA MONOGRAPHIE DU PRODUIT
AVERTISSEMENT NE DOIT PAS AJOUTER DE MEDICAMENT
SUPPLEMENTAIRE NE DOIT PAS ETRE MONTE EN SERIE
N'ADMINISTRER PAS SIMULTANEMENT AVEC LE SANG
N'EMPLOYER QUE SI LA SOLUTION EST LIMPIDE JETER TOUTE
PORTION INEMPLOYEE ADMINISTRER PAR UNE POMPE
D'INFUSION OU PAR UN DISPOSITIF IV A DEBIT MINUTIEUSEMENT
REGLE PRESSER ET INSPECTER LE SAC JETER EN CAS DE
FUITES ENTREPOSER ENTRE 15° ET 30°C

Viaflex® Plus PVC CONTAINER/CONTENANT DE PVC

Baxter   88-70-19-614
Baxter Corporation   NO NATURAL (LATEX) SANS LATEX
Toronto Ontario Canada RUBBER LATEX   NATUREL

0.8% Lidocaine HCl 2g (8 mg/mL)

FIGURE 10.1

Baxter Corporation, Toronto, Ontario.

Study the labels in Figure 10.2 and follow the example below, which illustrates the step-by-step approach to calculation.

Example: Order: heparin 12 units/kg/h; patient weighs 65.4 kg

Calculate the dose required: 12 units $\times$ 65.4 kg = 784.8 units/h. Round to 785 units/h.

Know the drug concentration. Read the label for heparin 20 000 units. The label states that 20 000 units is dissolved in 500 mL of 5% dextrose injection. The resulting concentration is 40 USP units/mL.

Calculate the rate of flow: $\dfrac{785 \text{ units/h}}{40 \text{ units/mL}} = 19.62$ mL/h. Round to 20 mL/h.

Validate: If 20 mL/h is the rate and each millilitre contains 40 units, then the rate is (20 $\times$ 40) 800 units/h. The order is for 785 units/h. **NOTE:** This rounding error is acceptable.

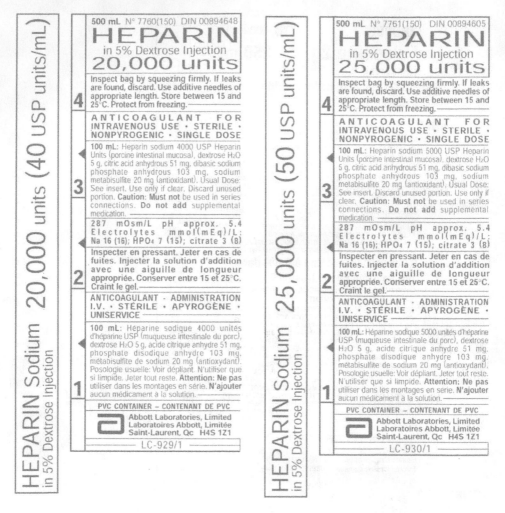

FIGURE 10.2
Reprinted with permission of Abbott Laboratories Limited, Montreal, Quebec.

▶ EXERCISE 10.2

This exercise presents a variety of more complex situations that have been taken from actual clinical settings in a large urban area and a rural hospital. Calculate the solutions. For each situation, write out each step of the calculation. Ask yourself: "What errors might occur in this calculation?" (Recall the advice in Module 9 to use failure mode and effects analysis to identify mistakes — *before* they happen.) Correct your answers by using the answer guide starting on page 192. (Value: 1 mark each)

Study the label in Figure 10.3 and answer questions 1 to 6.

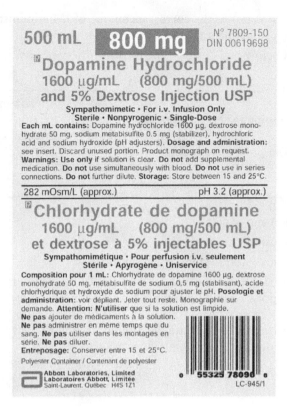

**500 mL   800 mg   N° 7809-150
DIN 00619698**

Dopamine Hydrochloride
1600 µg/mL   (800 mg/500 mL)
and 5% Dextrose Injection USP
Sympathomimetic • For i.v. Infusion Only
Sterile • Nonpyrogenic • Single-Dose
Each mL contains: Dopamine hydrochloride 1600 µg, dextrose mono-
hydrate 50 mg, sodium metabisulfite 0.5 mg (stabilizer), hydrochloric
acid and sodium hydroxide (pH adjusters). **Dosage and administration:**
see insert. Discard unused portion. Product monograph on request.
Warnings: Use only if solution is clear. **Do not** add supplemental
medication. **Do not** use simultaneously with blood. **Do not** use in series
connections. **Do not** further dilute. **Storage:** Store between 15 and 25°C.

282 mOsm/L (approx.)   pH 3.2 (approx.)

Chlorhydrate de dopamine
1600 µg/mL   (800 mg/500 mL)
et dextrose à 5% injectables USP
Sympathomimétique • Pour perfusion i.v. seulement
Stérile • Apyrogène • Uniservice
Composition pour 1 mL: Chlorhydrate de dopamine 1600 µg, dextrose
monohydraté 50 mg, métabisulfite de sodium 0,5 mg (stabilisant), acide
chlorhydrique et hydroxyde de sodium pour ajuster le pH. **Posologie et
administration:** voir dépliant. Jeter tout reste. Monographie sur
demande. **Attention: N'utiliser** que si la solution est limpide.
Ne pas ajouter de médicaments à la solution.
Ne pas administrer en même temps que du
sang. **Ne pas** utiliser dans les montages en
série. **Ne pas** diluer.
Entreposage: Conserver entre 15 et 25°C.
Polyester Container / Contenant de polyester

Abbott Laboratories, Limited
Laboratoires Abbott, Limitée
Saint-Laurent, Québec H4S 1Z1

0 55325 78090 0
LC-945/1

FIGURE 10.3
Reprinted with permission of Abbott Laboratories Limited, Montreal, Quebec.

1. What is the total volume contained in the product?
2. What is the total amount of drug (dopamine hydrochloride)?
3. What is the drug concentration in mcg/mL?
4. What is the IV solution?

For questions 5 and 6, use the formula below and the product in Figure 10.3.

$$\frac{\text{Amount required (mcg)} \times \text{Weight (kg)} \times 60 \text{ min/h}}{\text{Concentration (mcg/mL)}} = \text{Flow rate (mL/h)}$$

5. The order is for dopamine 8 mcg/kg/min. The patient weighs 178 lb. Calculate the rate of flow. Round to the nearest whole number.
6. The order is for dopamine 5 mcg/kg/min. The patient weighs 75 kg. Calculate the rate of flow. Round to the nearest whole number.
7. Order: fentanyl citrate 0.8 mcg/kg as premedication
   Supply: a 2-mL vial labelled "100 mcg"; therefore, the concentration is 50 mcg/mL
   The patient weighs 66 kg. Calculate the volume to administer. Round to the nearest tenth.
8. The order is for ceftriaxone 25 mg/kg IM for a 6-year-old child who weighs 24 kg. The vial label reads: "Rocephin (ceftriaxone sodium): to prepare low volume reconstitution for IM use, reconstitute with 1% lidocaine solution."

NOTE: This situation relates to the correct technique of IM administration for a child; please consult a fundamentals text for further information.

Read the label below and describe the reconstitution and calculate the volume to give.

Vial Size	Volume to Be Added to Vial (mL)	Approximate Available Volume (mL)	Approximate Average Concentration (g/mL)
1 g	2.2	2.8	0.35

9. Order: epinephrine 1 mg sc stat

   Supply: (1:1000 solution) 1 mg/mL

   Calculate the volume to administer for the stat dose.

10. The order is for ceftriaxone (Rocephin) 500 mg q2h IV by IVPB; infuse over 30 min. The 1-g vial instructions read: "To prepare for IV administration, add 9.6 mL of diluent to produce an approximate volume of 10.1 mL for an approximate average concentration of 0.1 g/mL." Calculate the amount to add to a 50-mL minibag to deliver the required dose.

Your Score:	/10	=	%

▶ EXERCISE 10.3

Complete the exercise without referring to the above text unless otherwise directed. Round answers as follows: for rate of flow of IV infusions, round to the nearest whole number; for parenteral doses, round to the nearest hundredth. Correct your answers by using the answer guide starting on page 192. (Value: 1 mark each)

The recommended dosage is gentamicin 1 mg/kg q8h. The drug is supplied in the following strength: each millilitre contains gentamicin 40 mg. Dosage reduction in renal impairment is made per Table 10.2. Answer questions 1 to 3.

TABLE 10.2 Dosing Schedule for Gentamicin

Approximate Creatinine Clearance Rate (mL/min/1.73 m²)	Percentage of Usual Adult Dose
> 100	100
70–100	80
55–70	65

Calculate the doses for the following people:

1. Mrs. Wong, age 81, weight 54.6 kg, creatinine clearance rate 67
2. Jacob, age 31, weight 220 lb., creatinine clearance rate 100
3. Madeline, age 9, weight 31 kg, creatinine clearance rate 75
4. Order: potassium phosphate monobasic 10 mmol IVPB bid
   Supply: 1.29 mmol/mL
   Calculate the volume of drug to add to the minibag.
5. The order is for calcium gluconate 0.1 mmol/kg/h given by IV over 10 h. The patient weighs 100 kg. You have a 10-mL ampule that contains 1 g (25 mmol of elemental calcium). Assume that you will add the drug to 500 mL of D5W and infuse over 10 h (i.e., 50 mL/h). Calculate the amount of calcium to add to the IV bag.

Study the label in Figure 10.1 (page 169) and answer questions 6 to 8.

6. Calculate the rate of flow in millilitres per hour to administer 2 mg/min of lidocaine. Round to the nearest whole number.
7. The IV is running at 40 mL/h. Does this exceed the recommended rate for lidocaine administration?
8. Calculate the rate of flow in drops per minute to administer 3.5 mg/min of lidocaine. Use a macrodrip set: 1 mL = 12 drops. Round to the nearest whole number.

Study the labels in Figure 10.2 (page 170) and answer questions 9 and 10.

9. Calculate the dose to deliver 12 units/kg/h for a patient weighing 74.8 kg.
10. Use the product labelled heparin 25 000 units. Calculate the rate of flow in millilitres per hour to deliver the dose in question 9. Validate your answer and assess the rounding error.

Your Score:	/10	=	%

▶ EXERCISE 10.4

Complete the exercise without referring to the above text. Round answers as follows: for rate of flow of IV infusions, round to the nearest whole number; for parenteral doses, round to the nearest hundredth. Correct your answers by using the answer guide starting on page 192. (Value: 1 mark each)

Order: ondansetron (Zofran) 8 mg IV q8h

Supply: a 4-mL vial labelled "2 mg/mL," with instructions to add to a 50-mL minibag and administer over 15 min

Answer questions 1 to 3.

1. Calculate the amount of drug to add to the minibag.
2. Calculate the rate of flow in millilitres per hour to deliver the drug.
3. Calculate the rate of flow in drops per minute using an IV set with a drop factor of 10.

An adolescent is admitted to the emergency department with severe bronchospasm. His weight is 45 kg. The orders are for stat IM Ventolin 8 mcg/kg followed by IV bolus of 4 mcg/kg over 2 to 5 min. Commence IV infusion 5 mcg/min. The drug is available in three concentrations:

- For IM injection: 0.5 mg/mL
- For IV bolus: 0.05 mg/mL
- For IV infusion: 1 mg/mL

Answer questions 4 to 10.

4. Calculate the dose for the stat IM injection.
5. Using the correct strength, calculate the volume for the IM injection.
6. Calculate the dose for the IV bolus.
7. Using the correct strength, calculate the volume for the IV bolus.
8. The instructions for the IV infusion are "add 5 mL to 500 mL." What is the resulting concentration of the solution?
9. Using the IV solution prepared in question 8, calculate the rate of flow in millilitres per hour to deliver the dosage.
10. The IV infusion has been running for 20 min. Calculate the total amount of Ventolin received by the patient, by all routes.

Your Score:	/10	=	%

▶ OPTIONAL ACTIVITY

Throughout this book, you have been encouraged to manage all situations involving calculations of medication doses with a systematic and consistent approach. This module has given you the opportunity to meet the challenges of more complex situations; however, the basic steps remain important. Always read the medication order and the label on the drug product very carefully. This activity presents labels of medications that are supplied in various strengths to illustrate the risks of error.

Complete the activity. Correct your answers by using the answer guide starting on page 192. (Value: 1 mark each)

Study the labels in Figure 10.4 and answer questions 1 to 5.

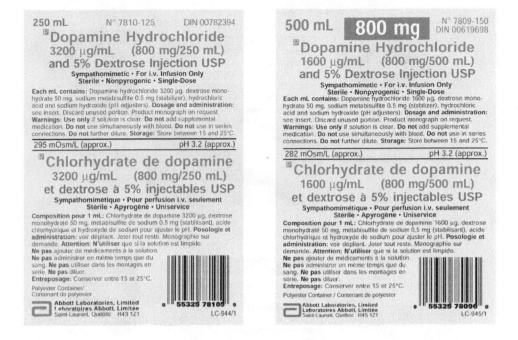

FIGURE 10.4
Reprinted with permission of Abbott Laboratories Limited, Montreal, Quebec.

1. What is the concentration of each product in micrograms per millilitre?
2. What is the solute in each of these products?
3. What is the solvent in each of these products?
4. If you intended to use the solution labelled "800 mg/500 mL" but used the solution labelled "800 mg/250 mL," what degree of error would occur? Would the patient receive double or half the intended dose?
5. What warnings are given on the labels?

Study the labels in Figure 10.5 and answer questions 6 to 10.

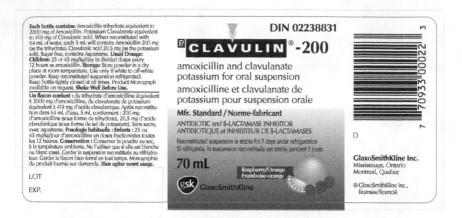

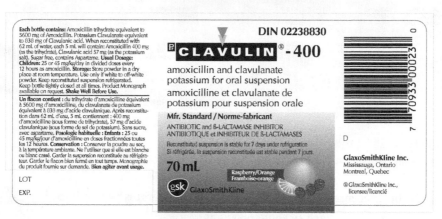

FIGURE 10.5
GlaxoSmithKline, Inc., Mississauga, Ontario.

6. Compare the strengths of the two products. Which drug preparation is the greatest strength?

7. What is the total amount of amoxicillin in the bottle of Clavulin-200?

8. What is the recommended dosage range for children?

9. Describe how to reconstitute each bottle.

10. What instructions are provided regarding storage and use?

Your Score:	/10	=	%

► CASE STUDIES

Study Box 10.2 and then answer questions 1 to 10. Correct your answers by using the answer guide starting on page 192. (Value: 1 mark each)

BOX 10.2 Epinephrine Hydrocloride (Adrenalin) Concentration

Prepare the appropriate concentration by mixing the indicated amount of drug in the volume of IV solution. Select the dose in micrograms per minute from the left column. Follow the line across the table to determine the rate of flow in millilitres per hour.

Dose (mcg/min)	1 mg/250 mL (4 mcg/mL)	4 mg/500 mL (8 mcg/mL)	2.5 mg/250 mL (10 mcg/mL)
0.5	7	4	—
1	15	8	6
2	30	15	12
3	45	23	18
4	60	30	24
5	75	38	30
6	90	45	36

The concentration of the epinephrine solution is 4 mcg/mL. State:

1. The number of mg in 250 mL of IV solution
2. The rate of flow necessary to deliver 2 mcg/min
3. How many micrograms are delivered in 15 min if the rate of flow is 45 mL/h
4. The concentration of the epinephrine solution in micrograms per millilitre if 4 mg were added to 500 mL
5. The flow rate required to deliver 1 mcg/min of the solution in question 4
6. How many micrograms per minute the patient is receiving if the IV pump is set at 23 mL/h

A 250-mL bag is labelled "1 mg epinephrine added."

7. What is the dose in micrograms per minute if the rate is 15 mL/h?
8. What rate is required to deliver 3 mcg/min?
9. The IV is running at 30 mL/h for 30 min. How much (total) epinephrine has the patient received?
10. The order states, "Run epinephrine at 4 mcg/min." The IV pump is set at 30 mL/h. *Is this correct?*

Read the following three case studies and answer questions 11 to 20. Refer to Table 10.3 and Boxes 10.3 to 10.5 on page 179 for available supply and for preparation of IV fluid. Correct your answers by using the answer guide starting on page 192. (Value: 1 mark each)

Mr. M., age 55, is admitted complaining of chest pain. Telemetry showed short runs of multifocal PVCs (premature ventricular contractions) followed by ventricular fibrillation; CPR was commenced and an IV was initiated (with a minidrip set). The orders are as follows:

lidocaine 100 mg IV bolus
lidocaine commenced 4 mg/min
pronestyl 1 g IV bolus
lidocaine drip discontinued
pronestyl drip at 4 mg/min
calcium gluconate 1 ampule

Calculate the following:

11. Lidocaine bolus
12. Lidocaine drip: describe the preparation
13. Lidocaine drip: state the flow rate
14. Pronestyl bolus
15. Pronestyl drip: describe the preparation
16. Pronestyl drip: state the flow rate

A middle-aged man in the coronary care unit (CCU) is monitored; he weighs 71 kg. An IV is running with a minidrip set and volumetric pump. Respiratory arrest and ventricular tachycardia occur. The orders are as follows:

lidocaine 100 mg IV bolus
xylocaine drip 1 mg/min
dopamine drip 3 mcg/kg/min
Lasix 20 mg IV bolus

17. Xylocaine drip: describe the preparation and state the flow rate.
18. Lasix bolus

Mrs. T. was admitted by ambulance to the CCU. She was short of breath and was experiencing retrosternal chest pain radiating to the jaw. The order is for Isuprel drip 2 mcg/min.

19. Isuprel drip: describe the preparation and state the flow rate.
20. State the flow rate to increase the drip to 2.5 mcg/min.

Your Score: /20   =   %

TABLE 10.3 Emergency Medications

Drug	Strength	Volume (ampule or vial)
dopamine HCl (Intropin)	40 mg/mL	5-mL ampule
furosemide (Lasix)	10 mg/mL	4-mL ampule
isoproterenol HCl (Isuprel)	1 mg/5 mL	5-mL ampule
lidocaine HCl (Xylocaine)	20 mg/mL	5-mL ampule
lidocaine HCl (Xylocaine)	1 g/50 mL	50-mL vial
procainamide HCl (Pronestyl)	100 mg/mL	5-mL ampule

BOX 10.3 Lidocaine (Xylocaine) Drip

Add 2 g to 500 mL D5W.

1 mg/min = 15 mL/h
2 mg/min = 30 mL/h
3 mg/min = 45 mL/h
4 mg/min = 60 mL/h

BOX 10.4 Procainamide (Pronestyl) Drip

Add 2 g to 500 mL for a concentration of 4 mg/mL.

1 mg/min = 15 mL/h
2 mg/min = 30 mL/h
3 mg/min = 45 mL/h
4 mg/min = 60 mL/h

BOX 10.5 Isoproterenol HCl (Isuprel) Drip

Add 2 mg to 500 mL IV solution for a concentration of 4 mcg/mL.

1 mcg/min = 15 mL/h
2 mcg/min = 30 mL/h
3 mcg/min = 45 mL/h
4 mcg/min = 60 mL/h

▶ POST-TEST

Instructions

1. Write the post-test without referring to any resources.

2. For each situation, write the problem and solution, and then validate your answer.

3. Round decimal numbers to the nearest hundredth unless otherwise indicated.

4. Correct the post-test by using the answer guide starting on page 192. (Value: 1 mark each)

1. An infant weighing 600 g is to receive gentamicin sulfate (Garamycin) 2.5 mg/kg by IV infusion q12h. The drug is supplied in a concentration of 10 mg/mL. Calculate the volume of drug to add to the IV fluid.

An infant weighing 11 lb. must receive a loading dose of aminophylline 7.5 mg/kg by IV infusion over 20 min. This is to be followed by maintenance doses of 0.5 mg/kg/h by continuous IV infusion. The drug is available in an ampule of 50 mg/5 mL. Answer questions 2 to 4.

2. Calculate the loading dose for the order above.

3. Calculate the amount of drug to add to a 25-mL IV minibag to produce a concentration of 1 mg/mL for the order above.

4. Calculate the rate of flow for the maintenance dose for the order above.

5. An isoproterenol drip is running at 1 mL/h and delivers 2 mcg/kg/min. The infant weighs 1265 g. How much drug does the infant receive each hour?

Use the formula below for questions 6 to 9.

Formula Statement for Mixing Dopamine Solution for Infants:

To make 50 mL of solution that provides 5 mcg/kg/min at a rate of 1 mL/h:

5 mcg × ____ kg × 60 min × 50 mL = ____ mcg dopamine in 50 mL of IV solution

____ mcg ÷ 40 000 mcg/mL = ____ mL dopamine

Dopamine Drip

Using the solution concentration determined above, adjust the IV rate in millilitres per hour as follows:

IV Rate	Dopamine Dosage
0.5 mL/h	2.5 mcg/kg/min
1 mL/h	5 mcg/kg/min
1.5 mL/h	7.5 mcg/kg/min

---

6. The infant weighs 790 g. The order is for dopamine 5 mcg/kg/min. Calculate the amount of dopamine to add to a 50-mL IV solution.

7. Determine the rate of flow from the chart on the next page.

8. State the IV rate necessary to deliver 2.5 mcg/kg/min.

9. The infant's weight is 1170 g. The order is for dopamine 7.5 mcg/kg/min. Determine the amount of dopamine required to prepare the solution.

Complete the following table. Calculate all orders using a macrodrip (10 gtts/mL). For each order, state the rate of flow of the IV solution and the amount of drug delivered per minute. Round drops per minute to the nearest whole number. Round other answers to the nearest hundredth. An example is done for you.

Order	Rate of Flow (gtts/min)	Amount of Drug Delivered per Minute
1000 mL with 20 mmol KCl over 8 h	$\dfrac{1000 \text{ mL}}{8 \text{ h} \times 60 \text{ min}} \times 10 \text{ gtts}$ $= 21 \text{ gtts/min}$	$\dfrac{20 \text{ mmol}}{8 \text{ h} \times 60 \text{ min}} = 0.04 \text{ mmol}$
500-mL IV bag with 3 g calcium gluconate to run over 10 h	(10)	(11)
pantoprazole (Pantoloc) 40-mg/100-mL bag over 5 h	(12)	(13)
1 000 000 units antibiotic in 25-mL bag to infuse in 20 min	(14)	(15)

Read the label on the IV bag. Use the formula statement and answer questions 16 to 18. Determine the rate of flow in millilitres per hour. Express as a whole number.

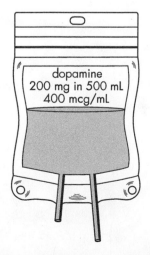

dopamine
200 mg in 500 mL
400 mcg/mL

16. Dopamine 3 mcg/kg/min for a patient weighing 52 kg

17. Dopamine 4 mcg/kg/min for a patient weighing 64 kg

18. The IV is running at 70 mL/h. The patient weighs 77 kg. How many micrograms per kilogram are delivered per minute?

19. State the concentration of medication in micrograms per millilitre if 400 mg of drug is added to 500 mL of IV solution.

20. Using an IV solution concentration of 1 mg/250 mL, calculate the rate of flow in millilitres per hour to deliver 3.5 mcg/min.

Your Score:	/20	=	%

Did you achieve 100%?

YES — Congratulations!

NO — Analyze your areas of weakness and review this module; then rewrite the post-test. If your score is still less than 100%, please seek remedial assistance.

Approximate Equivalents among Systems of Measurement

Apothecary	SI	Household
1 ounce (mass)	30 g	
1 grain	60 mg	
1 minum	—	1 drop
	5 mL	1 teaspoon
	15 mL	1 tablespoon
1 ounce (fluid)	30 mL	2 tablespoons
8 ounces	240 mL	1 measuring cup
	1 kg	2.2 pounds
	2.54 cm	1 inch

NOTE: For purposes of consistency, this book assumes that 1 cup equals 240 mL.

Temperature Conversions

Two facts should be kept in mind when converting temperatures between Fahrenheit and Celsius. First, the freezing point of water is 0°C and 32°F. Second, each degree Celsius is almost 2° Fahrenheit; in fact, 1°C equals 1.8°F exactly. You should always take these two facts into consideration when converting.

To convert degrees Celsius to degrees Fahrenheit:

1. Multiply by 1.8.
2. Add 32.

Example: 40°C = _____ °F

40 × 1.8 = 72

72 + 32 = 104

40°C = 104°F

Example: 36.4°C = _____ °F

36.4 × 1.8 = 65.52

65.52 + 32 = 97.52

36.4°C = 97.5°F
(rounded to tenth)

Example: −5°C = _____ °F

−5 × 1.8 = −9

−9 + 32 = 23

−5°C = 23°F

To convert degrees Fahrenheit to degrees Celsius:

1. Subtract 32.
2. Divide by 1.8.

Example: 105.3°F = _____ °C

105.3 − 32 = 73.3

73.3 ÷ 1.8 = 40.7

105.3°F = 40.7°C

Example: 98.6°F = _____ °C

98.6 − 32 = 66.6

66.6 ÷ 1.8 = 37

98.6°F = 37°C

Example: 19°F = _____ °C

19 − 32 = −13

−13 ÷ 1.8 = −7.2

19°F = −7.2°C

NOTE: One conversion is the reverse operation in the reverse order from the other.

Brand Names in Canada, Australia, and the United States

Generic	Canada	Australia	United States
acetaminophen	Atasol Tempra Tylenol	Paracetamol	Atasol Tempra Tylenol
acetylcysteine	Mucomyst	Mucomyst	Mucomyst
amikacin	Amikin	Amikin	Amikin
amphotericin B	Fungizone	Ambisome Fungilin Oral Fungizone	Amphocin Fungizone
ampicillin	Ampicin Penbritin	Alphacin Ampicyn Austrapen	Ampicin Penbritin
anileridine	Leritine	NA	NA
ASA	Aspirin Entrophen	Spren	Aspirin Entrophen
atorvastatin calcium	Lipitor	Lipitor	Lipitor
baclofen	(several others) Lioresal	Lioresal	Lioresal
bromocriptine mesylate	Parlodel	Parlodel	Parlodel
captopril	Capoten	Capoten	Capoten
carbenicillin disodium	Pyopen	NA	Geopen
carbidopa/ levodopa	Sinemet	Sinemet	Sinemet
cefaclor	Apo-Cefaclor Ceclor	Ceclor	Ceclor
cefazolin sodium (cephazolin [Aus])	Ancef Kefzol	Kefzol	Ancef Kefzol
cefotetan disodium	Cefotan	Apatef	Cefotan

(continued)

Generic	Canada	Australia	United States
ceftizoxime sodium	Cefizox	NA	Cefizox
ceftriaxone sodium	Rocephin	Rocephin	Rocephin
cefuroxime axetil (oral)	Ceftin	Zinnat	Ceftin
cefuroxime sodium (injectable)	Kefurox Zinacef	NA	Kefurox Zinacef
cephalexin	Keflex	Keflex	Keflex
cephalothin	Ceporacin	Keflin	NA
cyanocobalamin (injectable)	Cobalamin	Cytamen	several
dalteparin sodium	Fragmin	Fragmin	Fragmin
dexamethasone (oral)	Decadron Deronil Dexasone Oradexon	Decadron (injection)	Decadron Dexone Hexadrol
diclofenac sodium	Voltaren	Voltaren	Voltaren
digoxin	Lanoxin	Lanoxin	Lanoxicaps Lanoxin
digoxin immune Fab	Digibind	Digibind	Digibind Digidote
diltiazem	Cardizem	Auscard Cardizem	Cardizem
dimenhydrinate	Dramamine Gravol	Dramamine	Dramamine Gravol
diphenhydramine HCl	Benadryl	Benadryl	Benadryl
docusate sodium	Colace Soflax	Coloxyl	Colace Regulax
donepezil HCl	Aricept	Aricept	Aricept
dopamine	Intropin	dopamine	Intropin
epinephrine HCl	Adrenalin	Adrenaline	Adrenaline
erythromycin (several forms)	(several others) Erythromid	Erythrocin	(several others) E-Mycin
estrogens (conjugated)	Premarin	Premarin	Premarin

(continued)

Generic	Canada	Australia	United States
fentanyl citrate	fentanyl citrate	Sublimaze	Sublimaze
fentanyl (transdermal patch)	Duragesic	Duragesic	Duragesic
fluconazole	Diflucan	Diflucan	Diflucan
flumazenil	Anexate	Anexate	Romazicon
fluphenazine decanoate	Modecate	Anatensol Modecate	
fluphenazine HCl			Prolixin
furosemide (frusemide)	Lasix	Lasix	Lasix
gentamicin	Cidomycin Garamycin	Gentamicin	Garamycin
glyburide	Diaβeta (several others)	NA	Diaβeta
heparin sodium	Hepalean Heparin Leo	heparin injection	heparin injection
hydrochlorothiazide	HydroDiuril	Dichlotride	HydroDiuril
hydrocortisone hydrocortisone sodium succinate	Cortef Solu-Cortef	Hysone Solu-Cortef	Cortef Solu-Cortef
hydroxyzine	Atarax	NA	Hyzine Vistaril
indomethacin	Indocid	Indocid	Indocin
isoproterenol HCl	Isuprel	isoprenaline Isuprel	Isuprel
levothyroxine sodium	Eltroxin Synthroid	Oroxine	Eltroxin Synthroid
lidocaine HCl (lignocaine)	Xylocaine	Xylocaine	(several others) Dilocaine Xylocaine
lisinopril	Prinivil Zestril	Prinivil Zestril	Prinivil Zestril
lorazepam	Ativan	Ativan	Ativan
maprotiline	Ludiomil	NA	Ludiomil
meperidine	Demerol	pethidine	Demerol

(continued)

Generic	Canada	Australia	United States
methylprednisolone	Medrol		Medrol
methylprednisolone acetate	Depo-Medrol	Depo-Medrol	Depo-Medrol
methylprednisolone sodium succinate	Solu-Medrol	Solu-Medrol	Solu-Medrol
metronidazole	Flagyl	Flagyl	Flagyl Metro IV
misoprostol	Cytotec	Cytotec	Cytotec
morphine sulfate	Epimorph	Anamorph Kapanol	Astramorph PF
nadolol	Corgard	NA	Corgard
naloxone HCl	Narcan	Narcan	Narcan
naproxen	(several others) Naprosyn	Inza Naprosyn	(several others) Naprosyn
naproxen sodium	NA	Anaprox Naprogesix	NA
nitroglycerin	(several others)	(several others)	(several others)
nystatin	Mycostatin Nadostine Nilstat PMS-Nystatin	Mycostatin Nilstat	Mycostatin Nilstat Nystex
olanzapine	Zyprexa	Zyprexa	Zyprexa
pantoprazole	Pantoloc	Somac	Protonix
penicillin G potassium	NA	NA	Pfizerpen
penicillin G benzathine	Bicillin Megacillin	Bicillin	Bicillin Megacillin Wycillin
penicillin G procaine	Ayercillin		
penicillin V potassium	(several others) Ledercillin VK	(several others)	Pen-Vee K Ledercillin VK V-Cillin K
pericyazine	Neuleptil	Neulactil	NA
perphenazine	Trilafon	NA	Trilafon
phenobarbital	generic	phenobarbitone	Generic

(continued)

Generic	Canada	Australia	United States
phenytoin	Dilantin	Dilantin	Dilantin
potassium chloride	(several others) Slow-K Kay Ciel	(several others)	Kaon-CL (several others)
procainamide	Procan SR Pronestyl	Pronestyl	Procan SR Pronestyl
quinapril	Accupril	Accupril	Accupril
sulfasalazine	Alti-Sulfasalazine PMS-Sulfasalazine Salazopyrin	Salazopyrin	Azulfidine
theophylline	Theo-Dur Theolair	Theo-Dur	Theo-Dur Theolair
tinzaparin sodium	Innohep	NA	Innohep
trazodone HCl	Desyrel	NA	Desyrel
zopiclone	Imovane	Imovane	NA

(NA = not available)

Problem-Solving Approach

Although many readers and many instructors will be familiar with using proportion statements or cross multiplication to calculate doses, others may be more comfortable using problem-solving approaches. A simple and a more complex example are presented below.

The following problem-solving approach has been called *factor analysis, unit cancellation method,* and *dimensional analysis method.*

1. Write down what is given to you in the problem.
2. Place that quantity over 1.
3. Determine the relationship that is known; this is also called the *conversion factor.* At times the conversion factor is given to you in the problem; other times you are expected to know it.
4. Set up the problem statement as a fraction. Be sure to write the problem in such a way that the units are cancelled out.
5. Cancel the units: cancel the unit *lb.* in the numerator and the denominator, and you are left with the unit *kg* in the answer.
6. Solve.

Example: 80 lb. = x kg *or* Convert 80 lb. to kg.

Known: 80 lb.

Place quantity over 1: $\dfrac{80}{1}$

Conversion factor: 2.2 lb. = 1 kg

Problem statement: $\dfrac{80 \text{ lb.}}{1} \times \dfrac{1 \text{ kg}}{2.2 \text{ lb.}} = x \text{ kg}$

Cancel the units: $\dfrac{80 \text{ lb.}}{1} \times \dfrac{1 \text{ kg}}{2.2 \text{ lb.}} = \dfrac{80}{2.2} = 36.36 \text{ kg}$

80 lb. is equal to 36.36 kg.

---

1. Write down the problem.
2. Identify the conversion factor. In this problem, the conversion factor is given to you.
3. Set up the problem statement. What are you looking for? In this problem, you want to know how many millilitres to give per dose.
4. Cancel the units.
5. Solve.

Example: The order is to give morphine 8 mg IM. The medication is supplied in an ampule labelled "10 mg per mL."

Write the problem: x mL = 8 mg/dose

Conversion factor: 10 mg in 1 mL

Problem statement: $\dfrac{1 \text{ mL}}{10 \text{ mg}} \times \dfrac{8 \text{ mg}}{x \text{ mL}} = \dfrac{\text{mL}}{\text{dose}}$

Cancel the units: $\dfrac{1 \text{ mL}}{10 \text{ mg}} \times \dfrac{8 \text{ mg}}{x \text{ mL}} = \dfrac{8}{10} = 0.8 \text{ mL}$

Give 0.8 mL to deliver the ordered dose.

Answer Guide

NOTE: This answer guide is provided so you can check your answers to the self-assessment test, all exercises, and all post-tests. For those questions requiring basic arithmetic skills, only the answer is provided. For more complex skills, an example showing the process used to obtain the answer is provided. These examples are intended to assist you in analyzing any mistakes. To prevent a cumbersome answer guide, however, not all calculations are shown.

Self-Assessment Test

Part I: Whole Numbers
1. 1521
2. 2249
3. 626
4. 635
5. 131
6. 1189
7. 78
8. 13 776
9. 38 862
10. 48 642
11. 11 388
12. 4
13. 6
14. 5
15. 89

Part II: Fractions
1. $\dfrac{2}{3}$
2. $\dfrac{1}{2}$
3. $1\dfrac{1}{6}$
4. $1\dfrac{2}{3}$
5. $\dfrac{2}{55}$
6. $\dfrac{13}{60}$
7. $\dfrac{3}{8}$

8. $8\dfrac{3}{4}$
9. $\dfrac{23}{45}$
10. $\dfrac{5}{24}$
11. $\dfrac{3}{64}$
12. $2\dfrac{2}{15}$
13. $\dfrac{5}{16}$
14. $7\dfrac{1}{5}$
15. $\dfrac{7}{30}$
16. 1
17. $\dfrac{2}{3}$
18. $4\dfrac{1}{4}$
19. $\dfrac{3}{4}$
20. $1\dfrac{1}{2}$
21. 13
22. $5\dfrac{2}{5}$

23. $6\frac{5}{7}$

24. $14\frac{1}{3}$

25. $12\frac{2}{11}$

26. 6
27. 40
28. 18
29. 21
30. 16

31. $\frac{3}{8}$

32. $\frac{3}{7}$

33. $\frac{5}{28}$

34. $\frac{1}{3}$

35. $\frac{15}{32}$

36. mixed
37. improper
38. proper
39. proper
40. improper

41. $\frac{3}{9}$

42. $\frac{48}{16}$

43. $\frac{5}{25}$

44. no
45. yes

Part III: Decimal Numbers

1. 0.25
2. 0.5
3. 1.2
4. 1.1
5. 7.1
6. 9.74
7. 15.55
8. 2.01
9. 0.25
10. 0.2
11. 1
12. 8.01
13. 6.55
14. 8.02
15. 4.6
16. 6.6
17. 2.8
18. 1.4
19. 4.2
20. 0.07
21. 7
22. 500
23. 0.1
24. 50
25. 0.01
26. 30
27. 7.1
28. 2
29. 5.2
30. 2.2
31. 0.17
32. 1.6
33. 0.38
34. 0.75
35. 0.13

36. $\frac{7}{10}$

37. $\frac{8}{25}$

38. $1\frac{1}{4}$

39. $\frac{1}{50}$

40. $1\frac{1}{100}$

41. 0.001
42. 2.95

43. $\frac{9}{10}$

44. 90%
45. 1.75
46. 175%

47. $\dfrac{16}{25}$

48. 0.64

49. $\dfrac{1}{250}$

50. 0.4%

Module 1

Post-Test

1. 141
2. 205
3. 620
4. 776
5. 1771
6. 7475
7. 85
8. 23
9. $\dfrac{13}{14}$
10. $1\dfrac{5}{24}$
11. $1\dfrac{2}{3}$
12. $\dfrac{42}{55}$
13. $\dfrac{11}{18}$
14. $\dfrac{17}{21}$
15. $3\dfrac{1}{3}$
16. $\dfrac{25}{28}$
17. $\dfrac{1}{12}$
18. $\dfrac{1}{21}$
19. $1\dfrac{3}{10}$
20. $\dfrac{11}{24}$

21. $17\dfrac{2}{5}$
22. $\dfrac{7}{12}$
23. $\dfrac{3}{10}$
24. $\dfrac{1}{6}$
25. $\dfrac{1}{7}$
26. $\dfrac{1}{8}$
27. $\dfrac{27}{32}$
28. $3\dfrac{6}{7}$
29. $\dfrac{6}{25}$
30. 1
31. $1\dfrac{7}{9}$
32. $\dfrac{2}{11}$
33. $2\dfrac{2}{5}$
34. $1\dfrac{1}{6}$
35. $2\dfrac{2}{5}$
36. $\dfrac{2}{3}$
37. $1\dfrac{2}{3}$
38. $\dfrac{9}{14}$
39. $2\dfrac{2}{15}$
40. $1\dfrac{9}{10}$

41. $\dfrac{31}{9}$

42. $\dfrac{75}{8}$

43. $3\dfrac{3}{5}$

44. $2\dfrac{5}{7}$

45. 4

46. $28\dfrac{8}{9}$

47. $4\dfrac{2}{3}$

48. $1\dfrac{3}{5}$

49. 30
50. 36
51. 77
52. 15

53. $\dfrac{5}{12}$

54. $\dfrac{1}{4}$

55. 3

56. $\dfrac{1}{4}$

57. $\dfrac{1}{2}$

58. $1\dfrac{2}{3}$

59. $\dfrac{9}{8}$

60. $\dfrac{3}{14}$

61. $\dfrac{18}{42}$

62. $\dfrac{2}{12}$

63. $\dfrac{25}{80}$

64. $\dfrac{11}{12}$

65. 3.83
66. 10.31
67. 82.02
68. 10.39
69. 4.5
70. 2.7
71. 1.3
72. 2.5
73. 1.38
74. 22.44
75. 28.56
76. 11.84
77. 2
78. 6.3
79. 4.92
80. 6
81. 6.2
82. 81.7
83. 7.5
84. 7.9
85. 2.92
86. 3.45
87. 6.43
88. 182.61

89. $\dfrac{11}{50}$

90. 22%

91. $\dfrac{13}{25}$

92. 0.52
93. 0.2
94. 20%

95. $\dfrac{3}{5}$

96. 60%

97. $2\dfrac{3}{10}$

98. 230%
99. 1.125
100. 112.5%

Module 2

Exercise 2.1

1. 2:18 (or 1:9)
2. 18:20 (or 9:10)
3. 1 part drug to 1000 parts of solution
4. 25 units:1 tsp.
5. 12:48 (or 1:4)

Exercise 2.2

1. $\dfrac{1}{25}$
2. 0.04
3. 4%
4. 1:10
5. 0.1
6. 10%
7. 78:100 or 39:50
8. $\dfrac{78}{100}$ or $\dfrac{39}{50}$
9. 78%
10. 49:100
11. $\dfrac{49}{100}$
12. 0.49
13. 50:1
14. 50
15. 5000%

Exercise 2.3

1. Examples of solutions:

   Solve by using product of extremes = product of means:

   $3 \times x = 2 \times 12$

   $3x = 24$

   $x = \dfrac{24}{3} = 8$

   Validate by using cross multiplication.

   Solve by using cross multiplication:

   $\dfrac{2}{3} = \dfrac{x}{12}$

   $3 \times x = 2 \times 12$

   $3x = 24$

   $x = 8$

   Validate by using extremes = means.

2. 25
3. 21
4. 2

5.   1.5
6.   4
7.   0.35
8.   0.5
9.   0.25
10. 1
11. 4
12. 1080
13. 1
14. 0.5
15. 0.6

16. 16 scoops

Calculation by extremes = means:

6 (cups):4 (scoops) = 24 (cups):x (scoops)

$$6x = (4 \times 24) = 96$$
$$x = (96 \div 6) = 16$$

Validation by cross multiplication:

$$\frac{6}{4} = \frac{24}{x}$$
$$6x = (4 \times 24) = 96$$
$$x = (96 \div 6) = 16$$

17. 4 cups

Express

$1\frac{1}{2}$ as 1.5

Calculation by extremes = means:

1 (c milk):1.5(c mix) = x(c milk):6(c mix)

$$1.5x = 6$$
$$x = (6 \div 1.5) = 4$$

Validation by cross multiplication:

$$\frac{1}{1.5} = \frac{x}{6}$$
$$1.5x = 6$$
$$x = (6 \div 1.5) = 4$$

18. 15 gum

Calculation by extremes = means:

1 (gum):3 (mints) = x (gum):45 (mints)

$$3x = 45$$
$$x = (45 \div 3) = 15$$

Validation by cross multiplication:

$$\frac{1}{3} = \frac{x}{45}$$
$$3x = 45$$
$$x = (45 \div 3) = 15$$

19. 42 hot dogs

Calculation by extremes = means:

22 (children):33 (hot dogs)
   = 28 (children):x (hot dogs)
$22x = (33 \times 28) = 924$
$x = (924 \div 22) = 42$

Validation by cross multiplication:

$$\frac{22}{33} = \frac{28}{x}$$
$$22x = (33 \times 28) = 924$$
$$x = (924 \div 22) = 42$$

20. 8 cups
lime juice

Calculation by extremes = means:

1 (c. lime):3 (c. apple)
   = x (c. lime):24 (c. apple)
$3x = 24$
$x = (24 \div 3) = 8$

Validation by cross multiplication:

$$\frac{1}{3} = \frac{x}{24}$$
$$3x = 24$$
$$x = (24 \div 3) = 8$$

Exercise 2.4

1. A *ratio* is a relationship that exists between two quantities.
2. A *proportion* is the expression of two equal or equivalent ratios.
3. 234 males to 126 females (or 234:126)
4. 234 males to 360 total (or 234:360)
5. 10 crew to 350 passengers (or 1:35)
6. 25
7. 90
8. 7
9. 25
10. 4
11. 0.1
12. 123%
13. 0.335
14. $\dfrac{1}{2}$
15. The means are the numbers 3 and 4; the extremes are the numbers 2 and 6.

Post-Test

1. 45
2. 12
3. 25
4. 4
5. 4
6. 3
7. $\dfrac{1}{100}$
8. 0.01
9. 1%
10. $\dfrac{1}{5}$
11. 0.2
12. 20%
13. $\dfrac{1}{250}$
14. 0.004
15. 0.4%
16. 0.5
17. 165
18. 2000
19. 12.5
20. 7:5
21. 5:1
22. 17:3
23. 1.5
24. A *ratio* is a relationship that exists between two quantities.
25. *Proportion* is an expression of two equal or equivalent ratios.
26. 15
27. 15
28. 36
29. 1.5
30. 20

Module 3

Exercise 3.1

1. k
2. d
3. c
4. m
5. mc or μ
6. 1000
7. 0.000 000 001
8. 0.000 000 000 001
9. 0.001
10. 0.000 001
11. 0.01
12. 100
13. kilo, hecto, deca, deci, centi, milli, micro, nano

Exercise 3.2

1. m
2. 10 kg
3. 0.5 mL
4. L
5. 1000 mL
6. 0.5 L
7. 1050 mg
8. mL
9. 51 517
10. true

Exercise 3.3

1. 1000
2. 1000

3. 100
4. 1
5. 1 000 000
6. 0.25
7. 500
8. 200
9. 1000
10. 0.001

Exercise 3.4

1. 79.545 kg
2. 79.5 kg
3. 80 kg
4. 55 in.
5. 4 ft. 7 in.
6. 5 mL
7. 30 mL
8. 160 cm
9. 2 tsp.
10. 150 mL
11. 59.4
12. 15
13. 76.2
14. 9.5
15. 167.6
16. 60
17. 67.7
18. 250
19. 60.6
20. 8

Exercise 3.5

1. 1315 h
2. 0645 h
3. 0920 h
4. 2000 h
5. 2108 h
6. 2323 h
7. 2219 h
8. 0210 h
9. 3:57 P.M.
10. 9:30 P.M.
11. 2:15 P.M.
12. 11:59 P.M.
13. 12:05 A.M.
14. 3:00 A.M.
15. 10:30 P.M.
16. 11:00 A.M.
17. 7:50 P.M.
18. 5:05 P.M.
19. 2:16 P.M.
20. 1430 h

Exercise 3.6

1. 10
2. metre
3. kilogram
4. mole
5. k
6. h
7. dk
8. d
9. c
10. m
11. mc or μ
12. n
13. 1 kg equals 2.2 lb.
14. 5 mL
15. 2.54 cm

Post-Test

1. 10 000
2. 0.05
3. 250
4. 1250
5. 1000
6. 2000
7. 0.35
8. 150
9. 700 000
10. 102
11. 10
12. 77
13. 65
14. 66
15. 17
16. 960
17. 2160
18. 0715 h
19. 1530 h
20. 2200 h
21. metre, m
22. gram for metric; kg for SI, though g is most frequently used
23. mole, mol
24. 0.1
25. 0.01
26. 0.001
27. 0.000 000 001
28. 0.000 001

29. 1000
30. 1000
31. 1000
32. 0.01
33. 1000
34. 0.001
35. 0.25
36. 0.04
37. 0.2
38. 300
39. 100
40. 2.5

Module 4

Exercise 4.1

Part I

1. by intramuscular route every 3 to 4 hours as necessary
2. by mouth after meals three times a day
3. by mouth immediately and every 4 hours
4. by intravenous route 4 times a day
5. elixir 100 mg at bedtime
6. by subcutaneous route immediately
7. freely, as needed
8. drop
9. sublingual
10. suppository
11. after meals
12. tablet
13. twice a day
14. at bedtime
15. ointment
16. subcutaneous
17. extract
18. before meals
19. intramuscular
20. as much as required
21. with
22. immediately
23. solution

Part II

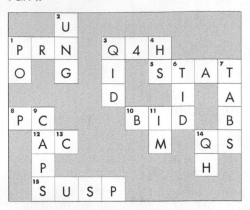

Exercise 4.2

1. solution
2. solute
3. solvent
4. b
5. a
6. gram
7. millilitre
8. millilitre
9. millilitre
10. weight-per-volume
11. volume-per-volume
12. 500 mg/mL
13. A *50% solution* means that 50 g of drug has been dissolved in 100 mL of solvent.
14. 5 g
15. One gram of drug (solute) has been dissolved in 10 000 mL of solvent. **NOTE:** Obviously the supply shown in Figure 4.6 is not the total volume; it is only 10 mL of the prepared solution.
16. 0.1 mg/mL
17. phenobarbital sodium
18. 30 mg/mL
19. 15 mg
20. 3% solution

Exercise 4.3

1. liquid
2. 10 mg/mL
3. Colace
4. docusate sodium
5. 2 mL (one to three times a day)
6. 30 mL
7. 50 000 iu
8. 10 000 iu/mL
9. heparin sodium
10. 5 mL

Exercise 4.4

1. Lioresal
2. baclofen
3. 10 mg/tab
4. 20 mg/tab
5. "Titration begins with 5 mg 3 times a day for 3 days, followed by increases to 10, 15, and 20 mg 3 times a day at 3-day intervals. Maximum dose should not exceed 80 mg daily (20 mg 4 times a day)."
6. 100 tablets
7. muscle relaxant, antispastic
8. Novartis Pharmaceuticals Canada Inc.
9. 33 days (with 1 tablet remaining)
10. product in Figure 4.11B (20 mg/tab)

Exercise 4.5

1. acetaminophen
2. relief of children's fever and pain
3. 80 mg/mL
4. 80 mg/mL
5. 32 mg/mL
6. 15 mL
7. 24 mL
8. 100 mL
9. 120 mg
10. A 0.5 mL graduated dropper
11. product in Figure 4.12C (160 mg/5 mL or 32 mg/mL)
12. Trianon Laboratories Inc.
13. 320 mg (10 mL × 32 mg/mL)
14. 6 doses (100 mL ÷ 15 mL = 6 doses with 10 mL remaining)

15. yes (According to the recommendations, the mother could choose between two doses: 1.5 or 2 tsp.)

Exercise 4.6

1. milligrams at bedtime as necessary
2. milliequivalents twice a day by intravenous route
3. milligrams orally three times a day
4. micrograms by intramuscular route
5. micrograms per kilogram by intravenous route immediately
6. volume-per-volume solution
7. weight-per-volume solution
8. 5 (g) in 100 (mL)
9. 10
10. 1:1000
11. 1:1000 = 1 mg/mL; 1:10 000 = 0.1 mg/mL
12. 0.6 mg (of 1:1000 strength)
13. 10 mg/mL
14. 80 mg/mL
15. 2.67 mEq/mL (tablespoon = 15 mL)

Post-Test

Part I

1. J
2. E
3. C
4. F
5. I
6. H
7. A
8. B
9. D
10. G

Part II

1. solution
2. Garamycin
3. gentamicin(e)
4. 40 mg/mL
5. intramuscular and intravenous
6. 20 mL

Part III
1. prednisone 30 mg orally for 3 days
2. digoxin 250 mcg orally daily
3. demerol 75 mg by intramuscular route every 3 to 4 hours as necessary
4. nitroglycerin spray by sublingual route as necessary
5. nifedipine tablet 20 mg orally twice a day
6. glycerin suppository per rectum as necessary
7. salbutamol inhaler 100 mcg/dose, 2 puffs every 4–6 hours
8. insulin 10 units by subcutaneous route immediately
9. antibiotic by intravenous piggyback
10. cough elixir as much as required

Part IV
1. b (10 000 units per mL)
2. 100
3. 1 g of drug is dissolved in 1000 mL of solution
4. 1 mg/mL

Part V
1. Heparin Leo
2. heparin sodium
3. Leo Laboratories Canada Ltd.
4. 10 000 i.u./mL
5. intravenous or subcutaneous

Module 5

Exercise 5.1

Calculations by cross multiplication and validations by extremes = means are shown.

1. $$\frac{0.125 \text{ mg}}{x \text{ tab}} = \frac{0.25 \text{ mg}}{1 \text{ tab}}$$

$$0.25x = 0.125$$
$$x = (0.125 \div 0.25) = 0.5$$

Give half a tab.

Validation:

$$0.125 \text{ mg}:0.5 \text{ tab} = 0.25 \text{ mg}:1 \text{ tab}$$
$$0.125 \times 1 = 0.5 \times 0.25$$
$$0.125 = 0.125$$

2. $$\frac{0.15 \text{ mg}}{x \text{ tab}} = \frac{0.05 \text{ mg}}{1 \text{ tab}}$$

$$0.05x = 0.15$$
$$x = (0.15 \div 0.05) = 3$$

Give 3 tabs.

Validation:

$$0.15 \text{ mg}:3 \text{ tabs} = 0.05 \text{ mg}:1 \text{ tab}$$
$$0.15 \times 1 = 3 \times 0.05$$
$$0.15 = 0.15$$

3. $$\frac{0.015 \text{ g}}{x \text{ tab}} = \frac{0.005 \text{ g}}{1 \text{ tab}}$$

$$0.005x = 0.015$$
$$x = (0.015 \div 0.005) = 3$$

Give 3 tabs.

Validation:

$$0.015 \text{ g}:3 \text{ tabs} = 0.005 \text{ g}:1 \text{ tab}$$
$$0.015 \times 1 = 3 \times 0.005$$
$$0.015 = 0.015$$

4. $$\frac{0.1 \text{ mcg}}{x \text{ tab}} = \frac{0.05 \text{ mcg}}{1 \text{ tab}}$$

Validation:

$$0.05x = 0.1$$
$$x = (0.1 \div 0.05) = 2$$

$$0.1 \text{ mcg}{:}2 \text{ tabs} = 0.05 \text{ mcg}{:}1 \text{ tab}$$
$$0.1 \times 1 = 2 \times 0.05$$

Give 2 tabs.

$$0.1 = 0.1$$

5. $$\frac{12.5 \text{ mg}}{x \text{ tab}} = \frac{50 \text{ mg}}{1 \text{ tab}}$$

Validation:

$$50x = 12.5$$
$$x = (12.5 \div 50) = 0.25$$

$$12.5 \text{ mg}{:}0.25 \text{ tab} = 50 \text{ mg}{:}1 \text{ tab}$$
$$12.5 \times 1 = 0.25 \times 50$$

Give a quarter tab.

$$12.5 = 12.5$$

Exercise 5.2

1. Use Lotensin 20-mg tabs and give 1 tab *or* use Lotensin 10-mg tabs and give 2 tabs.
2. Give 1 tab Voltaren 25 mg and 1 tab Voltaren 50 mg *or* give 3 tabs Voltaren 25 mg.
3. Use Lioresal 10 mg; break 1 tab in half and give $1\frac{1}{2}$ tabs.
4. Give 1 tab Anafranil 25 mg and 2 tabs Anafranil 50 mg *or* give 5 tabs Anafranil 25 mg.
5. Give 1 tab Anafranil 25 mg and 1 tab Anafranil 50 mg *or* give 3 tabs Anafranil 25 mg.
6. 1.5 tabs
7. 2 tabs
8. 0.5 tab
9. 1.5 tabs
10. 2 tabs
11. 1 tab of 10 mg and 1 tab of 20 mg *or* 3 tablets of 10 mg
12. 0.5 tab
13. 2 tabs
14. Break tablet in half and in half again. Give a quarter tab.
15. 2 tabs

Exercise 5.3

1. 0.125 mg = 125 mcg; give 1 tab
2. 0.5 g = 500 mg; give 2 tabs
3. 0.25 mg = 250 mcg; give 1 tab
4. 0.45 g = 450 mg; give 3 caps
5. 1 g = 1000 mg; give 4 tabs

Exercise 5.4

1. Ceclor
2. cefaclor
3. 250 mg/5 mL and 375 mg/5 mL
4. To reconstitute the Ceclor 250 suspension: invert bottle and tap to loosen powder, add 90 mL of water in two parts, and shake well after each addition. To reconstitute the Ceclor BID suspension: invert bottle and tap to loosen powder, add 42 mL of water in two parts, and shake well after each addition.

5. Give 2.5 mL.
6. 250 mg (1 tsp. = 5 mL)
7. 1500 mg (or 1.5 g); this does not exceed the maximum dose of 2 g/day
8. Each dose is 375 mg; give 5 mL.
9. 27 mL
10. Ceclor 250 (It contains 7.5 g, whereas the Ceclor BID contains only 5.25 g.)

Exercise 5.5

You should be able to locate the information on the labels in the module. Of interest, note that the label in Figure 5.1 does not have a trade name. It is manufactured by Trianon under the generic name acetaminophen. Note that some labels provide only adult doses (see Figure 5.2), and others state "not recommended for use in patients under 16 years of age" (see Figure 5.3). Some provide storage precautions such as "protect from heat and humidity" (see Figure 5.4) and others provide more specific information such as "store between 2°C and 30°C" (see Figure 5.5). Some labels do not provide the concentration per 1 mL; for example, the Ceclor labels state the concentration per 5 mL.

Exercise 5.6

1. The error was in the conversion from grams to milligrams.

Calculation:
$0.3 \text{ g} = 300 \text{ mg}$

$100 \text{ mg:1 tab} = 300 \text{ mg:}x \text{ tab}$

$100x = 300$

$x = (300 \div 100) = 3$

Give 3 tabs.

Validation:

$$\frac{100 \text{ mg}}{1 \text{ tab}} = \frac{300 \text{ mg}}{3 \text{ tabs}}$$

$100 \times 3 = 1 \times 300$

$300 = 300$

2. The wrong operation was performed.

Calculation:

$$\frac{\text{dose}}{\text{supply}} = x \text{ tab}$$

$$\frac{2.5 \text{ mg}}{1 \text{ tab}} = \frac{5 \text{ mg}}{x \text{ tab}}$$

$2.5x = 5$

$x = (5 \div 2.5) = 2$

Give 2 tabs.

Validation:

$2.5 \text{ mg:1 tab} = 5 \text{ mg:2 tabs}$

$2.5 \times 2 = 1 \times 5$

$5 = 5$

3. The conversion from milligrams to grams was not performed.

Calculation:
$2500 \text{ mg} = 2.5 \text{ g}$

$$\frac{1 \text{ g}}{1 \text{ tab}} = \frac{2.5 \text{ g}}{x \text{ tab}}$$

$1x = 2.5$

$x = 2.5$

Give 2.5 tabs.

Validation:
$1 \text{ g:1 tab} = 2.5 \text{ g:2.5 tabs}$

$2.5 = 2.5$

4. The ratios were not set up in a consistent order.

Calculation:

$15 \text{ mg}:5 \text{ mL} = 30 \text{ mg}:x \text{ mL}$

$15x = 150$

$x = (150 \div 15) = 10$

Give 10 mL.

Validation:

$$\frac{15 \text{ mg}}{5 \text{ mL}} = \frac{30 \text{ mg}}{10 \text{ mL}}$$

$15 \times 10 = 5 \times 30$

$150 = 150$

5. The arithmetic was performed incorrectly.

Calculation:

$$\frac{0.25 \text{ mg}}{1 \text{ tab}} = \frac{0.125 \text{ mg}}{x \text{ tab}}$$

$0.25 \times 0.5 = 1 \times 0.125$

$x = (0.125 \div 0.25) = 0.5$

Give a $\frac{1}{2}$ tab.

Validation:

$0.25 \text{ mg}:1 \text{ tab} = 0.125 \text{ mg}:0.5 \text{ tab}$

$0.25x = 0.125$

$0.125 = 0.125$

Case Study

1.
Generic Name	Trade Name
levothyroxine sodium	Eltroxin
levothyroxine sodium	Synthroid
digoxin	Lanoxin
furosemide	Lasix
indapamide	Lozide
omeprazole	Losec

2.
Drug	Available Strengths
Lanoxin	0.25 mg; 0.125 mg; 0.0625 mg
Lasix	20 mg; 40 mg; 80 mg
Synthroid	0.05 mg; 0.1 mg; 0.15 mg; 0.025 mg
Eltroxin	300 mcg; 50 mcg

3. Give 1 tab of 80-mg Lasix.
Give 1 tab of 0.25-mg and 1 tab of 0.125-mg digoxin *or* give 3 tabs of 0.125-mg strength.
Give 3 tabs of 0.025-mg Synthroid.

4. Give 1 tab of 40-mg Lasix.
Give 1 tab of 0.25-mg digoxin.
Give 3 tabs of 0.025-mg Synthroid.

5. 0.15 mg; 0.1 mg; 0.05 mg;
0.025 mg. **NOTE:** If you are unsure about the relative size of decimal numbers, then write them in a column and compare:
0.150
0.100
0.050
0.025

6. day 1: 3 tabs of 20 mg
   day 2: 4 tabs of 20 mg
   day 3: 3 tabs of 20 mg
   NOTE: The order for 40 mg is to be given at bedtime.
7. Give 1 tab of 2.5 mg.
8. One tablet of Eltroxin 300 mcg is the most accurate and is simple to administer; the alternative choice is 3 tabs of 0.1-mg Synthroid, but it is less desirable to give 3 tablets.
9. Synthroid: 1 tab of 0.05 mg
   Synthroid: 2 tabs of 0.025 mg
   Eltroxin: 1 tab of 50 mcg
   Use of either Synthroid 0.05-mg tab or Eltroxin 50-mcg tab would be most desirable.
10. 0.4375 mg
11. 0.25 mg = 250 mcg
    0.125 mg = 125 mcg
    0.0625 mg = 62.5 mcg
    NOTE: With this conversion, the comparative strengths are more obvious.
12. Give 2 tabs of 40 mg *or* give 4 tabs of 20 mg *or* give 2 tabs of 20 mg plus 1 tab of 40 mg.
13. Give 1 tab of 0.1-mg Synthroid.
14. Give 1 tab of 0.125-mg Lanoxin.
15. Give 1 tab of 20-mg Losec.

Post-Test

1. 2 caps
2. 4 caps (2 × 2 = 4)
3. 2 tabs
4. 56 tabs (2 × 4 × 7)
5. 1 tab (125 mcg = 0.125 mg)
6. 2 tabs
7. 2 tabs
8. half a tab
9. 6 mg
10. 12 mL
11. 10 mL
12. 15 doses
13. 3900 mg (2 × 6 × 325)
14. 3.9 g
15. 1 tab (0.15 mg = 150 mcg)
16. Convert order: amount of acetaminophen in 2 tablets is (320 mg × 2) 640 mg. Amount of acetaminophen elixir to deliver 640 mg is 20 mL.
17. Convert order: amount of codeine in 2 tablets is (30 mg × 2) 60 mg. Amount of codeine syrup to deliver 60 mg is 12 mL.
18. Give 1 tab of 100 mg plus 1 tab of 60 mg plus 1 tab of 15 mg.
19. Give 3 tabs of 0.0625 mg *or* 1 tab of 0.125 mg and 1 tab of 0.0625 mg.
20. 22.5 mL
21. 3 tabs
22. 5 mL
23. 800 000 units

24. 200 mg
25. 38.97 mg
26. 1.44 mEq
27. Give 1 tab of 5 mg and 1 tab of 10 mg.
28. Voltaren
29. diclofenac sodium
30. 150 mg
31. morning and/or evening, preferably at mealtimes
32. Give 1 tab of 75 mg *or* give 1 tab of 50 mg plus 1 tab of 25 mg.
33. Break a 10-mg tab; give half a tab.
34. Give 3 tabs of 50 mg plus 1 tab of 25 mg.
35. Give 6 tabs of 50 mg.
36. 2.5 g
37. Lotensin
38. benazepril hydrochloride
39. 2 tabs
40. 4 tabs

Module 6

Exercise 6.1

1. (a) 1 mL (or 1 cc)
   (b) 0.65 mL

2. (a) 2.5 mL or $2\frac{1}{2}$ mL

   (b) 2.1 mL
3. (a) 3 mL (or 3 cc)
   (b) 1.8 mL
4. (a) 1 mL (or 1 cc)
   (b) 0.72 mL

5. (a) 2.5 mL or $2\frac{1}{2}$ mL

   (b) 1.5 mL

Exercise 6.2

1. 10 000 units:1 mL = 7500 units:x mL
   10 000x = 7500
   $x = (7500 \div 10\ 000) = 0.75$
   Give 0.75 mL.
2. Known ratio: 50 mg:1 mL
   Unknown ratio: x mg:1.5 mL
   50:1 = x:1.5
   $x = 75$
   The answer is 75 mg.

3. $\dfrac{250\ \text{mg}}{1\ \text{mL}} = \dfrac{400\ \text{mg}}{x\ \text{mL}}$

   250x = 400
   $x = (400 \div 250) = 1.6$
   Give 1.6 mL.

Validation: $250:1 = 400:1.6$
$400 = 400$

4. 1.5 mL
5. 0.8 mL
6. Convert: $200 \text{ mg} = x$ units
$(200 \times 1600 = 320\,000)$
Solve: $400\,000 \text{ units}:1 \text{ mL} = 320\,000 \text{ units}:x \text{ mL}$
$400\,000x = 320\,000$
$x = (320\,000 \div 400\,000) = 0.8$
Give 0.8 mL.

Validation:

$$\frac{400\,000 \text{ units}}{1 \text{ mL}} \times \frac{320\,000 \text{ units}}{0.8 \text{ mL}}$$

$320\,000 = 320\,000$

7. 0.5 mL
8. 0.8 mL
9. 0.6 mL
10. 1.5 mL

Exercise 6.3

1. 0.46 mL
2. 2.4 mL
3. 1.2 mL
4. 0.78 mL
5. 32 units (or 0.32 mL)
6. 0.85 mL
7. 54 units (or 0.54 mL)
8. 0.13 mL

Exercise 6.4

1. 9.3 mL
2. 1.3 mL
3. 3.8 mL
4. 2 mL
5. 1.3 mL
6. 250 000 IU
7. 200 000 IU
8. 350 000 IU
9. 1.9 mL sterile water for injection
10. 1 h
11. 1.6 mL
12. IM and IV
13. penicillin G sodium
14. 3.1 mL sterile water for injection
15. 1 million IU/mL
16. 24 h at room temperature and 7 days refrigerated
17. 1 mL
18. 0.4 mL

19. 0.7 mL
20. 1.5 mL

Exercise 6.5

1. no; 0.25 mL
2. 1 mL is needed, not 1 ampule. The ampule may contain more than 1 mL.
3. no; 0.5 mL
4. no; 4.3 mL
5. yes

Exercise 6.6

1. Garamycin
2. gentamicin
3. 800 mg
4. 1.6 mL
5. intramuscular and intravenous
6. 1 mL (of 10 000 IU) and 3.8 mL (of 25 000 IU)
7. 10 000 IU/mL and 25 000 IU/mL
8. intravenous or subcutaneous

9.
$$\frac{25\ 000\ IU}{1\ mL} = \frac{2500\ IU}{x\ mL}$$

$25\ 000x = 2500$
$x = (2500 \div 25\ 000) = 0.1$
Give 0.1 mL.

Validation:
25 000 IU:1 mL = 2500 IU:0.1 mL
2500 = 2500

10. The product labelled 25 000 IU/mL is much more concentrated than the product labelled 10 000 IU/mL. The degree of error = (25 000 ÷ 10 000) = 2.5 times the desired dose.
11. 1 mg/mL
12. Each millilitre contains atropine sulfate, an isotonicity agent, and a pH adjuster.
13. IM, IV, and SC
14. 0.6 mg:x mL = 1 mg:1 mL
$x = 0.6$
Give 0.6 mL.

15.
$$\frac{0.6\ mg}{x\ mL} = \frac{1\ mg}{1\ mL}$$

$x = 0.6$
Give 0.6 mL.

Case Study

1. 0.6 mL
2. 1 mL
3. 1 mL
4. 1 mL
5. 10 mL

Post-Test

1. 250 mg/mL
2. 1 mL
3. 14:00 h
4. 1000 mg
5. 0.7 mL
6. 1.5 mL
7. 0.75 mL
8. 0.75 mL
9. 5.3 mg
10. 0.83 mL
11. 23.4 mg
12. Product A has the greatest concentration. It has 400 mcg/mL, whereas product B has 20 mcg/mL.
13. Use product A; give 0.5 mL.
14. Use product A. The required dose is 85 mcg; therefore, give 0.21 mL.
15. Compare: 0.5 mL of product A = 200 mcg, whereas 0.5 mL of product B = 10 mcg. The error is twentyfold.
16. 1.2 mg
17. 0.1 mL
18. 1.25 mL
19. 0.4 mL
20. 3 mL

Module 7

Exercise 7.1

1. $\dfrac{1000 \text{ mL}}{(8 \times 60 \text{ min})} \times 10 \text{ gtts/mL} = 21 \text{ gtts/min}$

2. $\dfrac{1000 \text{ mL}}{(x \times 60 \text{ min})} \times 60 \text{ gtts/mL} = 50 \text{ gtts/min} = 20 \text{ h}$

3. $\dfrac{500 \text{ mL}}{(4 \times 60 \text{ min})} \times 10 \text{ gtts/mL} = 21 \text{ gtts/min}$

4. $\dfrac{500 \text{ mL}}{(4 \times 60 \text{ min})} \times 60 \text{ gtts/mL} = 125 \text{ gtts/min}$

5. $\dfrac{x \text{ mL}}{(1 \times 60 \text{ min})} \times 15 \text{ gtts/mL} = 25 \text{ gtts/min}$

$\dfrac{15x}{60} = 25$

$x = 100$
The rate is 100 mL/h.

Validation:

$$\frac{100 \text{ mL}}{60 \text{ min}} \times 15 \text{ gtts/mL} = 25 \text{ gtts/min}$$

$$25 = 25$$

6. 125 mL/h

7. $\dfrac{100 \text{ mL}}{60 \text{ min}} \times 10 \text{ gtts/mL} = 17 \text{ gtts/min}$

8. 20 h

9. $\dfrac{50 \text{ mL}}{20 \text{ min}} \times 10 \text{ gtts/mL} = 25 \text{ gtts/min}$

10. 563 mL

11. $\dfrac{50 \text{ mL}}{60 \text{ min}} \times 60 \text{ gtts/mL} = 50 \text{ gtts/min}$

12. $\dfrac{100 \text{ mL}}{60 \text{ min}} \times 10 \text{ gtts/mL} = 17 \text{ gtts/min}$

The answer is *no* because 20 gtts/min is too *fast*.

13. $\dfrac{400 \text{ mL}}{50 \text{ mL/h}} = 8 \text{ h}$

14. $\dfrac{500 \text{ mL}}{(3 \times 60 \text{ min})} \times 15 \text{ gtts/mL}$

$$= 42 \text{ gtts/min}$$

15. $\dfrac{250 \text{ mL}}{x \text{ min}} \times 10 \text{ gtts/mL} = 125 \text{ gtts/min}$

$$x = 20 \text{ min}$$

Exercise 7.2

1. 48 min
2. Add 3.8 mL of sodium chloride injection or sterile water for injection to a 500-mg vial.
3. approximately 2.2 mL
4. 1.1 mL
5. 1.5 mL
6. Garamycin
7. 40 mg/mL
8. 20 mL
9. Add 2 mL of drug to the minibag.
10. 30 gtts/min

Exercise 7.3

1. Add 3.1 mL sterile water for injection.
2. 1 million IU/mL
3. 24 h at room temperature and 7 days refrigerated

4. $\dfrac{\text{Dose}}{\text{Supply}} \times \text{Vehicle} = \text{Amount to administer}$

$$\frac{750\ 000\ \text{IU}}{1\ 000\ 000\ \text{IU}} \times 1\ \text{mL} = 0.75\ \text{mL}$$

Withdraw 0.75 mL.

5. Validation:
   750 000 IU:x mL = 1 000 000 IU:1 mL
   1 000 000 x = 750 000

   $$x = \frac{750\ 000}{1\ 000\ 000} = 0.75$$

6. Add 0.75 mL of penicillin to a 50-mL minibag.
   Concentration: 750 000 IU in 50 mL
   = 15 000 IU/mL
7. 17 gtts/min
8. Add 3.5 mL sterile water for injection.
9. 250 mg/mL
10. 1 h
11. 400 mg:x mL = 250 mg:1 mL
    $250x = 400$
    $x = (400 \div 250) = 1.6$
    Withdraw 1.6 mL.

12. $\dfrac{400\ \text{mg}}{x\ \text{mL}} = \dfrac{250\ \text{mg}}{1\ \text{mL}}$

    $250x = 400$
    $x = (400 \div 250) = 1.6$
13. Add 1.6 mL of reconstituted drug solution to a 50-mL minibag.
    Concentration:
    400 mg in 50 mL = 8 mg/mL
14. 30 gtts/min
15. 2.5 mL/h

Exercise 7.4

1. Add 1.9 mL sterile water for injection to yield about 2 mL. Add another 3 mL of sterile water for injection to further dilute to 5 mL.
2. Withdraw 2 mL.
3. 13 gtts/min
4. Fragmin
5. dalteparin sodium
6. 25 000 IU/3.8 mL
7. 3.8 mL

8.   10 000 IU/mL
9.   1 mL
10. 2500 IU/0.2 mL
11. 0.2 mL
12. 0.5 mL
13. 0.08 mL
14. 0.05 mL
15. 25 000 IU/mL (see Figure 7.8*A*); 2500 IU/0.2 mL (see Figure 7.8*C*); 10 000 IU/mL (see Figure 7.8*B*)

Case Studies

1.   21 gtts/min
2.   17 gtts/min
3.   3000 mg (or 3 g)
4.   receives 6 infusions of 50-mL with medication = 300 mL; primary infusion at 125 mL for 21 h (24 h less the 3 h of medication infusions) = 2625 mL. The total volume infused over 24 h is 2925 mL.
5.   150 mL of NS (3 infusions of 50-mL minibags)
6.   primary infusion of D5W at 100 mL for 21.5 h (24 h less 2.5 h of medication infusions) = 1250 mL *plus* 2 infusions of 50-mL minibags = 2250 mL
7.   1.5 g × 2 doses = 3 g
8.   80 mg × 3 doses = 240 mg
9.   50 gtts/min
10. 500 mg/200 mL = 2.5 mg/mL

Post-Test

1. $\dfrac{500 \text{ mL}}{3 \times 60 \text{ min}} \times 10 \text{ gtts/mL} = 28 \text{ gtts/min}$

2.   60 min
3.   1330 h
4.   1500 mL
5.   480 mL
6.   Use 2 vials. Add 20 mL sterile water to each vial, dissolve completely, and add both vials.
7.   17 gtts/min
8.   63 × 2 = 126 mg of sodium
9.   Add 7 mL.
10. 21 gtts/min
11. Each 10-mL ampule contains (10 × 0.1 mg) 1 mg; therefore add 10 ampules to the 100 mL bag.
12. 20 gtts/min
13. The minimum concentration requires 180 mL of IV fluid; add 12 mL of Septra to a 200-mL bag.
14. 22 gtts/min
15. 200 gtts/min
16. 0.8 mL
17. 5 mg (or 0.2 mL)
18. Add 6 vials (2 mL in each vial and 20 mg in each vial).
19. 20 mL/h to deliver 8 mg/h

20. Add 5 mL.
21. Add 6 mL.
22. Add 0.75 mL.
23. Add 3 mL.
24. 1500 mg
25. 94 mL/h

Module 8

Exercise 8.1

Part I

1. 0.8 mL
2. 0.4 mL
3. 1.2 mL
4. No. Both drugs are supplied in single-dose ampules.

Part II

5. (a) 8 units
   (b) no insulin
   (c) 7 units
   (d) 10 units
   (e) 4 units
   (f) 4 units
6. The syringe should be shaded at 10 units.
7. 8 units ac lunch, none at supper, and 7 units hs = total of 15 units
8. 10 units ac lunch, 4 units ac supper, and 4 units hs = total of 18 units

Part III

9. (a) 18
   (b) 10
   (c) 10
   (d) regular
   (e) 18
   (f) NPH
   (g) 28
10. (a) Humulin-N
    (b) Humulin-R
    (c) 8
    (d) Humulin-R
    (e) 25
    (f) Humulin-N
    (g) 33

Exercise 8.2

1. the 25 000-IU bag because it has a concentration of 50 units/mL
2. 50 kg
3. (a) 12 mL/h
   (b) 11 mL/h

NOTE: For answers 4 to 7, a base rate of 11 mL/h according to answer 3(b) is chosen.

4. Add 2 mL/h = 13 mL/h
5. Add 1 mL/h = 14 mL/h
6. 14 mL × 50 IU = 700 units/h
7. (a) 0915 to 1315 = 4 h × 11 mL = 44 mL
    1315 to 1915 = 6 h × 13 mL = 78 mL
    The total IV fluid intake is
    122 mL.
    (b) 122 mL × 50 IU/mL = 6100 IU.
8. 5 mg
9. Give 1 tablet of 5 mg and half a tablet of 5 mg (1.5 tabs total).
10. 920 IU/h

Exercise 8.3
1. 3.75 mL
2. 6 mL
3. Give 6 mL of 1-mg/mL solution *or* give 0.6 mL of 10-mg/mL solution or give 1 mL of 1-mg/mL solution plus 1 mL of 5-mg/mL solution.
4. Mix 75 parts enteral solution with 25 parts water.
   The volume of the total solution is (50 mL/h × 4) 200 mL (75% of 200 = 150 mL enteral solution; 25% of 200 = 50 mL water).
5. 10 mL

Exercise 8.4
1. Withdraw the medication in the multi-dose vial first to avoid contaminating the remaining drug product.
2. Withdraw the clear (short- or rapid-acting) insulin first to avoid contaminating it with the modified (cloudy, longer-acting) insulin.
3. Use a 1-mL syringe.
4. sliding scale insulin protocol
5. 5 units
6. The physician should be notified.
7. No insulin should be administered at that time.
8. 0.35 mL
9. The correct volume is 0.55 mL. If the colleague rounded to the nearest tenth, then 0.6 mL would be correct. However, it is more accurate to give 0.55 mL (5500 units) than to give 0.6 mL (6000 units). For this drug product, even a small volume contains a significant amount of medication.
10. 7000 units

Case Study
1. Give 0.5 mL.
2. 20 units/mL
3. 50 mL/h
4. Rate change: increase by 10 mL/h to 60 mL/h
5. 1200 units/h
6. no change
7. Stop the infusion for 30 min; reduce the rate by 5 mL/h to 55 mL/h.

8.   The table below illustrates the steps in the calculation.

Time	Number of Units	Total Units
0800 h (day 1)	5000 (bolus)	5 000
0815 h – 1615 h	1000 units × 8 h	8 000
1615 h – 0815 h (day 2)	1200 units × 16 h	19 200
	Total	32 200

9.   The total amount of heparin received was 32 200 units.
      The rate of flow was 8 h at 50 mL/h and 16 h at 60 mL/h; the total amount
      infused was (8 × 50) + (16 × 60) 1360 mL.
10.   The 24-h period required 3 infusions.

Post-Test

1.   no insulin
2.   8 units
3.   no insulin
4.   8 units
5.   5 units
6.   11 mL/h
7.   21 mL/h
8.   36 mL/h × 50 units/mL = 1800 units/h
9.   No. The rate is 36 mL/h (the maximum rate).
10.   850 units/h
11.   14 875 units
12.   1.49 mL
13.   0.1 mL
14.   0.5 mL
15.   17 460 IU
16.   0.7 mL
      NOTE: Do not include the zero after the 7; write as 0.7 according to the rules
      for SI decimal numbers.
17.   0.35 mL
18.   20 IU/mL
19.   87.3 kg × 200 IU = 17 460 IU in 24 h = 728 IU/h
20.   36 mL/h
21.   Use one 10-mg/mL ampule and one 50-mg/mL ampule for a total volume of
      2 mL of meperidine. Alternatives: use 0.8 mL of the 75-mg/mL ampule *or* use
      0.6 mL of the 100-mg/mL ampule. The first option does not waste any medica-
      tion; however, the final volume in the syringe may be too much for a comfortable
      injection.
22.   0.6 mL
23.   2.6 mL, 1.4 mL, *or* 1.2 mL
      NOTE: Most references indicate a maximum of 3 mL for an IM injection. A
      decision must be made regarding the size of the patient. It is beyond the scope
      of this book to teach administration techniques.
24.   0.38 mL (38 units)
25.   0.15 mL (15 units)

Module 9

Pediatric Case Study

1. q8h or tid
2. 115 mg
3. 0.9 mL
4. 3.8 mL diluent added to 500-mg vial
5. 32 lb. = 14.5 kg; 25 mg × 14.5
   = 363.75 mg daily
6. 363.75 ÷ 3 equal doses = 121.25 mg each dose
7. 115 mg is slightly less than
   121 mg; explanation: the table uses approximations
8. 0.7 mL

Exercise 9.1

1. 4 mg × 20 kg = 80 mg
2. 80 mg ÷ 4 doses = 20 mg
3. 5 mg × 51.2 kg = 256 mg — within the recommended range
4. 34.3 lb = 15.59 kg; 15.59 kg × 4 mg ÷ 4 doses = 15.6 mg
5. range is (17 kg × 0.5 mg) 8.5 mg to (17 kg × 1 mg) = 17 mg — within the
   recommended range
6. 0.43 mL
7. 0.27 mL
8. Yes, within recommended range. (The recommended dose is 0.01 mL/kg,
   which is equivalent to 10 mcg/kg and the solution is 1 mg/mL or
   1000 mcg/mL; therefore, 0.01 mL = 10 mcg.)
9. Give 0.15 mL.
10. The syringe should be shaded at 0.15 mL.

Exercise 9.2

1. range is (25 × 15) 375 mg to (50 × 15) 750 mg
2. 3 doses/d, each dose = 125 mg to 250 mg
3. Add 5 mL to vial labelled 250 mg. Add entire contents to small-volume chamber,
   and fill chamber to 20 mL.
4. 60 gtts/min
5. The range is 246–410 mcg.
6. 0.49 mL
7. 0.82 mL
8. 0.33 mL
9. 12.5 mg/h
10. 20 mL/h

Exercise 9.3

1. 1.5 tabs
2. 1.5 mL
3. 4 mL
4. 1.4 mL
5. 7.5 mL
6. half a tab
7. Give 8 tabs of 5 mg *or* give half a tab of 50 mg plus 3 tabs of 5 mg.

8.   10 mL
9.   11.9 mg
10. 0.25 mL

Exercise 9.4

1.   The 25-mg and the 50-mg tabs can be crushed.
2.   Give 1 tab of 25 mg for each dose.
3.   150 mg
4.   Initially, 25–50 mg three times daily, depending on the severity of the condition. For maintenance, 25 mg three times daily or the minimum amount to provide continuous control of symptoms. Once a maintenance dose of 75 mg/d has been established with Voltaren enteric-coated tablets, a once-daily dose of Voltaren SR 75 mg may be substituted, taken morning or evening.
5.   25% × 50 mg = 12.5 mg; give 0.25 mL
6.   1 mg/10 mL or 0.1 mg/mL
7.   10 mL
8.   2 mL
9.   1 mg
10. 2.5 mL

Exercise 9.5

1.   3.2 mL
2.   10 mg × 17 kg = 170 mg. If using the product in Figure 9.6A, give 2.1 mL. If using the product in Figure 9.6B, give 5.3 mL.
3.   37 lb. = 16.8 kg × 15 mg = 252 mg. If using the product in Figure 9.6A, give 3.2 mL. If using the product in Figure 9.6B, give 7.9 mL.
4.   For the product in Figure 9.6A: the recommended dosage is 3 mL (240 mg) every 4 hours, up to 5 times a day or as directed by the physician. (Recall that the term *dosage* refers to a system of doses; that is, the dose and the frequency of administration — see Module 5.) For the product in Figure 9.6B, the recommended dosage is either 1 tsp. (5 mL) or 1.5 tsp. (7.5 mL) every 4 hours up to 5 times a day, or as directed by the physician.
5.   Mrs. Johnson should use one of the calibrated devices (see Figure 9.1) to ensure accuracy. **NOTE:** These devices are available at drugstores and are usually provided with the drug product. The client should consult the pharmacist.
6.   Clavulin
7.   amoxicillin and clavulanic acid
8.   25 mg/mL (125 mg amoxicillin in 5 mL)
9.   50 mg/mL
10. 37.1 kg × 13.3 mg/kg = 493.43 mg. The volume required if using the product in Figure 9.7A is 20 mL. The volume required if using the product in Figure 9.7B is 10 mL.

Geriatric Case Study

1.   Anafranil
2.   1 tab
3.   Lioresal
4.   half a tab
5.   15 mg

6. Combine 30 mL of Maalox Regular Suspension with 15 mL of lidocaine 2% viscous solution.
7. 100 mg every other day
8. single dose for days 1 to 3: 5 mg; single dose for day 4: 10 mg
9. number of tabs for each dose for days 1 to 3: half a tab; number of tabs for each dose for day 4: 1 tab
10. total daily dosage for days 1 to 3: 15 mg; total daily dosage for day 4: 30 mg

Post-Test

1. 6.6 mL (30 mg $\times$ 16.4 kg = 492 mg divided into 3 doses = 164 mg)
2. 3.2 mL
3. 0.19 mL (0.015 mg $\times$ 3.2 kg = 0.048 mg)
4. 34 kg $\times$ 0.01 mg = 0.34 mg; within recommended range
5. 5.8 mL
6. 0.78 mL
7. 0.2 mL
8. 560 mg
9. 93.33 mg
10. 0.75 mL
11. 0.26 mL
12. received 60 $\times$ 6 mg = 360 mg; maximum recommended dose not to exceed (7.2 kg $\times$ 65 mg) 468 mg; did not exceed recommended dose
13. quarter tab
14. 10 005 mg
15. 1 mL IM
16. half a tab of 4 mg
17. 2 tabs of 0.5 mg
18. 1 tab of 0.5 mg
19. 11 mg
20. 2 mL
21. 1 mL
22. 0.3 mL (Remember to convert milligrams to micrograms.)
23. 56.3 mL
24. no (SR = slow release)
25. half a tab

Module 10

Exercise 10.1

1. 18.75 mL $\times$ 200 mg/mL = 3750 mg
2. 75 mL
3. 200 mL
4. 15 min
5. 133 gtts/min
6. The concentration is 40 mL (200 mg/mL) in 1 L: 40 $\times$ 200 $\div$ 1000 = 8 mg/mL.

    If 1600 mL is absorbed over 16 h, then assume 375 mL is absorbed in 6 h.

    375 mL $\times$ 8 mg/mL = 3000 mg or 3 g

    Therefore, 3 g have been delivered.

7. $$\frac{11.25 \text{ mL} \times 200 \text{ mg}}{40 \text{ mL D5W}} = 56.25 \text{ mg/mL}$$

8. 38 tabs × 0.25 mg × 0.8 = 7.6 mg. Since 1 vial binds 0.5 mg, 16 vials are required.

9. Convert micrograms to milligrams. 30 tabs × 0.125 mg × 0.8 = 3 mg; 6 vials required

10. 50 tabs × 0.0625 mg × 0.8 = 2.5 mg; 5 vials required

Exercise 10.2

1. 500 mL
2. 800 mg
3. 1600 mcg/mL
4. 5% dextrose
5. 178 lb. = 80.9 kg

$$\frac{8 \text{ mcg} \times 80.9 \text{ kg} \times 60 \text{ min/h}}{1600 \text{ mcg/mL}} = 24 \text{ mL/h}$$

6. $$\frac{5 \text{ mcg} \times 75 \text{ kg} \times 60 \text{ min/h}}{1600 \text{ mcg/mL}} = 14 \text{ mL/h}$$

7. 1.1 mL
8. The dose required is 25 mg × 24 kg = 600 mg. Add 2.2 mL of 1% lidocaine to the vial for a concentration of 350 mg/mL (or 0.35 g/mL). Use 1.71 mL to deliver the dose.

9. 1 mL
10. Add 5 mL to 50 mL.

Exercise 10.3

1. 1 mg × 54.6 kg = 54.6 mg; 54.6 mg × 65% = 35.5 mg. The drug concentration is 40 mg/mL. Use 0.89 mL.

2. 220 lb. = 100 kg; 1 mg × 100 kg × 100% = 100 mg. The drug concentration is 40 mg/mL. Use 2.5 mL.

3. 1 mg × 31 kg = 31 mg × 80% = 24.8 mg. The drug concentration is 40 mg/mL. Use 0.62 mL.

4. 7.75 mL
5. dose required: 0.1 mmol × 100 kg = 10 mmol/h; volume per hour = 50 mL, therefore, 1 mmol/50 mL is required (equals 10 mmol/500 mL). Add 4 mmol to the 500-mL bag. **NOTE:** The drug concentration is 25 mmol/10 mL or 2.5 mmol/mL.

6. 15 mL/h
   Validation: 15 mL/h would deliver 15 × 8 mg/mL = 120 mg/h; this is equal to 120 mg ÷ 60 min = 2 mg/min.

7. 40 mL/h would deliver 40 × 8 mg = 320 mg/h. This exceeds the limit of 300 mg/h.

8. 5 gtts/min
9. 898 units/h
10. 18 mL/h
    Validation: 18 mL/h will deliver 18 × 50 units/mL = 900 units/h. This is an acceptable rounding error.

Exercise 10.4

1. Add 4 mL to the 50-mL minibag.
2. 200 mL/h
3. 33 gtts/min
4. 360 mcg (8×45)
5. 0.72 mL
6. 180 mcg
7. 3.6 mL
8. 5 mg in 500 mL = 0.01 mg/mL or 10 mcg/mL
9. 30 mL/h
   Validation: 30 mL = 30×10 mcg = 300 mcg/h = $300 \div 60 = 5$ mcg/min)
10. 640 mcg (IM 360 + IV bolus 180 + IV infusion of 5 mcg/min $\times$ 20 min = 100 mcg)

Optional Activity

1. The product labelled "800 mg/500 mL" contains 1600 mcg/mL.
   The product labelled "800 mg/250 mL" contains 3200 mcg/mL.
2. dopamine hydrochloride
3. 5% dextrose solution
4. double the intended dose
5. "Use only if solution is clear. Do not add supplemental medication. Do not use simultaneously with blood. Do not use in series connections. Do not further dilute."
6. Clavulin-400
7. 2800 mg
8. 25 or 45 mg/kg/d in divided doses every 12 h
9. For Clavulin-200, add 64 mL of water; for Clavulin-400, add 62 mL of water.
10. "Store powder in a dry place at room temperature. Use only if white to off-white powder. Keep reconstituted suspension refrigerated. Keep bottle tightly closed at all times."

Case Studies

1. 1 mg
2. 30 mL/h
3. 3 mcg/min $\times$ 15 = 45 mcg
4. 8 mcg/mL
5. 8 mL/h
6. 3 mcg/min
7. 1 mcg/min
8. 45 mL/h
9. $2 \times 30 = 60$ mcg
10. No. It should be set at 60 mL/h.
11. Give 5 mL of the 20-mg/mL strength.
12. Add 2 g to a 500-mL bag (use 2 vials of 50 mL).
13. 60 mL/h
14. Use 2 ampules of 5 mL (10 mL = 1000 mg).
15. Add 2 g (4 ampules of 5 mL) to 500 mL.
16. Infuse at 60 mL/h.
17. Add 2 g (2 vials of 50 mL) to 500 mL; infuse at 15 mL/h.

18. Give 2 mL of 10 mg/mL strength.
19. Add 2 mg (or 2 ampules of 5 mL) to 500 mL; infuse at 30 mL/h.
20. 2 mcg/min = 30 mL/h; 3 mcg/min = 45 mL/h; 2.5 mcg/min is midway between 30 and 45 = 37.5 (or 38) mL/h.

Post-Test

1. Convert 600 g = 0.6 kg; dose 2.5 mg × 0.6 kg = 1.5 mg. Add 0.15 mL.
2. Convert 11 lb. = 5 kg; 7.5 mg × 5 kg = 37.5 mg by IV infusion.
3. Add 25 mg. Available supply is 50 mg/5 mL; add 2.5 mL to the 25-mL minibag.
4. dose required = 0.5 mg × 5 kg = 2.5 mg/h = 2.5 mL/h
5. 2 mcg × 1.265 kg × 60 min = 151.8 mcg/h
6. 5 mcg × 0.79 kg × 60 min × 50 mL = 11 850 mcg; 11 850 mcg/40 000 mcg = 0.296 (approximately 0.3) mL
7. 1 mL/h
8. 0.5 mL/h
9. 7.5 mcg × 1.17 kg × 60 min × 50 mL = 26 325 mcg; 26 325 mcg/40 000 mcg = 0.66 mL

10. $$\frac{500 \text{ mL} \times 10 \text{ gtts}}{10 \text{ h} \times 60 \text{ min}} = 8 \text{ gtts/min}$$

11. $$\frac{3 \text{ g}}{10 \text{ h}} = \frac{3000 \text{ mg}}{10 \times 60} = 5 \text{ mg/min}$$

12. $$\frac{100 \text{ mL} \times 10 \text{ gtts}}{5 \text{ h} \times 60 \text{ min}} = 3 \text{ gtts/min}$$

13. $$\frac{40 \text{ mg}}{5 \text{ h} \times 60 \text{ min}} = 0.13 \text{ mg/min}$$

14. $$\frac{25 \text{ mL} \times 10 \text{ gtts}}{20 \text{ min}} = 13 \text{ gtts/min}$$

15. $$\frac{1 \text{ 000 000 units}}{20 \text{ min}} = 50 \text{ 000 units/min}$$

16. $$\frac{3 \text{ mcg} \times 52 \text{ kg} \times 60 \text{ min}}{400 \text{ mcg/mL}} = 23 \text{ mL/h}$$

   Validation: 23 mL/h and 400 mcg/mL
   23 × 400 = 9200 mcg/h
   Divide by patient's weight = 176.9 mcg/kg/h
   Divide by time = 2.95 mcg/kg/min (acceptable rounding error)

17. $$\frac{4 \text{ mcg} \times 64 \text{ kg} \times 60 \text{ min}}{400 \text{ mcg/mL}} = 38 \text{ mL/h}$$

Validation: 38 mL/h and 400 mcg/mL
38 × 400 = 15 200 mcg/h
Divide by patient's weight = 237.5 mcg/kg/h
Divide by time = 3.96 mcg/kg/min (acceptable rounding error)

18. $$\frac{x \text{ mcg} \times 77 \text{ kg} \times 60 \text{ min}}{400 \text{ mcg/mL}} = 70 \text{ mL/h}$$

$x = 6$
6 mcg/kg delivered per minute

19. Convert: 400 mg = 40 000 mcg

$$\frac{40\ 000 \text{ mcg}}{500 \text{ mL}} = 800 \text{ mcg/mL}$$

20. Concentration is 1 mg/250 mL = 1000 mcg/250 mL = 4 mcg/mL;
3.5 mcg/min = 3.5 × 60 = 210 mcg/h

$$\frac{210 \text{ mcg/h}}{4 \text{ mcg/mL}} = 52.5 \text{ mL/h}$$

Validation: 52.5 mL/h delivers 52.5 × 4 mcg = 210 mcg/h;
210 mcg/h = 210 ÷ 60 min = 3.5 mcg/min

Index